Hindrances

Cheryl Saler

PublishAmerica
Baltimore

First printing

ISBN: 1-4241-2312-7
PUBLISHED BY PUBLISHAMERICA, LLLP
www.publishamerica.com
Baltimore

Printed in the United States of America

About the Author

My name is Cheryl Saler. This book is a true story of what happened to my family and me. You will learn the story of what happens to a brain tumor survivor. As I wrote this book it brought back so many memories that were horrible and wonderful. The marvel of it all is I am one of the few people who survive the ordeal without any disabilities. The emotional scars run very deep and the hurt I inflicted upon my family also is something that I hope would never have to endure again. I have a very large scar that goes across my head and an indentation from where my skull had to be replaced with titanium. Through the process I learned just how wonderful love and life are, not that I didn't know before but it became intensified.

The most important people I should thank are: First is my husband, Bob, he was there for me and still is. He was my "Rock" in this whole endeavor. Also: my two daughters, Dana & Aja. They also gave me support and helped in so many ways. Bob, Dana & Aja were my reason to fight to come back. I wasn't done being a wife and mother, a human being. My family gave me more than I could ever give to them.

Next I would like to thank my Mother. She stayed with us and helped with the recovery and gave us strength to get through it. Without her help we would have a much more difficult time. No matter how old we get, we will always need our mothers.

Next and just as important, I would like to thank the doctors who worked so hard to save my life and my physical abilities. They were wonderfully skilled people who let me continue to live.

Also, I would like to thank the rest of my family who did what they could to help. Their concern and kind words helped more than I can ever tell them.

Just as important as anything from this whole ordeal I would like to thank God. He allowed me to stay here on earth with my family. Without his help and guidance the ordeal would have been much worse.

1.
Obstacles

The sight in my left eye just kept on fading. The eye doctor told me in May it was a vitamin deficiency from when I had shingles in my side. That sounded believable to a point, although my shingles were nowhere near my face, the vitamin deficiency sounded correct as I was worn out. At least it wasn't macular degeneration that can happen to people who reach their forties.

Bob and I spent hours working on the new English garden he created for my birthday and Mothers day gift. We were enjoying spending time outside planning, talking and just being together.

Suddenly in July he had to stop helping and start relaxing. He lifted a box incorrectly at work and hurt his back again. This has been an ongoing problem and this time the twist and lift were just right to make problems for him. Trip after trip to the doctors and many hours of consultation let us know he would need another surgery. It was up to his timing and when he wanted it taken care of.

The summer went by in a hurry and September quickly closed in on us. We were picking beans off the lattice fencing in the garden and I suddenly noticed I could not differentiate the greens in my left eye to tell what was bean or plant. I would close my right eye and try to see out of just the left and it would all go black and I couldn't see at all out of it. When I would look out of both eyes it was if there was a cataract in the way. The next day I was making French toast and could not tell where the white of my counter and the white of my dish ended. I could see the creamy eggs in the middle and not the counter and dish. A horrible chill went up my spine. My sight was fading, what was wrong with me? Did the eye doctor know what he was talking about? The very next day I called another eye doctor at the clinic I normally went to. It would take two weeks for an appointment to be open. Until then a waiting game would begin. I tried hard to concentrate on the current situation and my husband's back. I worried he too would have something go terribly wrong with that. He had another appointment with his spinal doctor and it was evident he would need another surgery. He chose October 1st. Until that time it would be a waiting game for him, try to relax and live with as little pain as possible. The medications weren't much help; he still limped and was bent over in pain.

Finally the anticipated eye doctor Appointment day came. The fear was great that Bob went with me to help calm my nerves. He too was worried as to what was happening to me. Was he going to have a blind wife?

Was it a side effect of Laser Surgery on our eyes? We all four had that done the year before and we all had a new found 20/20 vision. All those years of glasses and contacts were over. It was quite an adjustment. No more groveling for glasses in the morning to see the clock, or the endless hours spent trying to get the contacts clean and comfortable to wear. We sat there silently after I checked in and waited for them to call my name. I suddenly felt a strong sense of comfort and let out a big sigh. Bob reached over and squeezed my hand. "It will be ok, honey" he tried to reassure me. I tried to smile and just said, "Her first name is Dana, like our daughter, I can feel she will take care of me." Somehow deep inside I knew she was going to find out what the problem was.

She was very kind. I filled her in on the last few months. I let her know about the vision correction. She informed me they had done a very good job and my lenses were just fine. The sight test has shown my right eye to be 20/20 and the left eye was basically horrible. The vision kept on going blurry then it would black out. The doctor kept quiet, a deafening quiet. Then she began with lights and drops and never said another word for over 15 minutes. Suddenly the chills hit again and she saw the goose bumps on my arms. "Please try not to be alarmed, I need to order further tests." She was very reassuring in her explanations. "First we are going to start with a visual field test. On the same day you come in we are going to have you take blood tests to check your thyroid and pituitary glands." Often those glands cause sight trouble for women in my age group. Sometimes with the "change" coming this happens. Oh for the love of being forty something!

Bob looked like he was napping when I came out of the back from testing. He had almost dropped off to sleep from waiting for over an hour. "Wow, they really tested you didn't they?" I grabbed his hand and started to walk with him out of the clinic. The arrangements for the visual field test were made while I talked to the doctor. "I need to have more tests, but the good news is my right eye is fine." My hand grew very tight in his. He has so much to worry about with his upcoming surgery and so did I. We had to tell the girls their father needed surgery again. "Honey, I promise to help you with the surgery and recovery, what happens after that I will need your help." His blue eyes grew to a deeper blue as they always do when his is deep in thought. "We are going to get through this, it's all my fault," he continued. "I wish I had never said we are so lucky to not have anything bad happen in our life and how lucky we are, it's a curse." My heart sank, lower than I had been feeling about the events that were happening. "You are not responsible, the blame goes nowhere, it's out of our control this time." After we got in the car I began to tell him about the visual field tests and thyroid and pituitary tests that were to be taken. As usual he listened to me carry on about the reassuring doctor and how I liked her and felt confident she can help. As we were arriving home we agreed to talk to the girls about his surgery and not let them know at this time I was in trouble. One parent for them to worry about at this time seems cruel enough to do to them. Without any prognosis it would seem senseless. I made him promise to keep my secret and let them think the lightning bolt headaches were from stress.

The girls came for dinner that Friday night and brought the boyfriends along too. We laughed and joked around all evening. Then the other shoe fell. We informed them about the surgery for their father on October 1. Both girls got a little teary eyed. "Now ladies," Bob said, "I have had this surgery before and it worked for 6 years didn't it?" They both agreed. "Oh Dad," Dana said, " First that weird stomach virus that didn't go away for three months now this." We all agreed, it has been a rough 2002 so far. Bob and I glanced at each other without a word. "I know the doctor will do a good job, we have complete faith in him. Now let's just enjoy this evening," he told Dana and Aja. Everyone agreed while the questions were asked and we made jokes again about the last surgery. We decided this time there would be no bell in the bedroom for Bob to ring when he wanted something, last surgery he rang it to be funny.

The next evening we went to the Paul McCartney concert. It was the most fun we had together in a very long time. Bob and I went out to eat at a restaurant he had never been to. Dana took me there for Mothers day the year before. The staff is paid to insult people and the food is great too. We giggled like children all the way through dinner. Then it was off to the concert. The music was so wonderful; it took until the fifth song until we realized we were actually sitting there listening to Paul McCartney. The arena reflected the sound so you could feel it rumble through your body. We were again trapped in our youth remembering how we loved to go to concerts and simply enjoy the musicians. I kept closing my eyes and reminiscing and trying to stop the headache from the strain of trying to see it clearly. Once a chill went up my spine again and the consideration of blindness consumed my soul. Quickly I shook the thoughts away and started to concentrate on the music again. The two and a half hour concert went by too fast. "Hello, goodbye" rang through our heads as well as the other wonderful songs played that evening.

Sunday morning is never a sleep in day as it should be. Angel and Winston, our two Springer spaniels want us up. They are so used to eating by six a.m. that trying to appease them in any other way is hopeless.

The morning review in the paper about the concert was a rave. We sat and reminisced and decided we need to do more of that kind of fun in our lives again. After the morning paper, the usual Sunday brunch was made and we started in on planning the rest of the day. The phone rang and my brother Paul said he was bringing up a load of wood for the fireplace in the afternoon. That was also an excuse because he was also very concerned about what was happening to us. He knew about the doctor appointments and was helping us keep it from our mothers. His pick up truck was full of firewood, we made Bob coach and only lift the small pieces. His daughter Diana came and helped also. She started asking questions about my headaches trying to compare them to hers. It was getting harder and harder to keep the secret, and then it happened again, another lightning bolt headache and I had to sit down. Paul thought of a quick excuse to send Diana into the house and then turned and asked when I was going to do something more about this problem. I filled him in on the tests so far and changed the subject to the concert we had seen the night before. Out of the corner of my right eye I could see Bob touch his shoulder as if to say "back off." Paul nodded and agreed with Bob. I looked at them both and said, "You should do that from my left side and I won't see what you're both up to." Those tears were tough to swallow, that look of concern from my brother and husband hurt as bad as the fear inside me.

My mother called that evening. "Have you had your eye exam yet?" I filled her in without letting on what exactly was happening. Then I filled her in on the surgery that Bob was going to have. She would be busy with my Aunt coming from England at that time, which was actually a good thing. My other Aunt had liver cancer and she was coming to see her for what she thought would be the last time. These two women are my deceased father's sisters. How I wished I could have Dad to talk to again. But would I be able to tell him what was happening to me? Being the youngest in the family of five children it would have been too much for him to handle. He cared very deeply for all of us. I just wished he could be there to hold my mom's hand and help her. As usual, when mom calls we talk for an hour. When the call was over Bob knew how hard it was to not let on what was happening and reassured me I did the right thing by not telling my mother.

The next morning came with great anticipation. The visual field day was here. Never had one before and didn't know what to expect. I sat in front of a white bowl that flashed little lights. A clicker was put in my hand to push every time I saw a light. Right eye was good again. Left eye, "Where are the dots of light?" I blinked and blinked trying to see them. My eye began to throb trying so hard to see out of it. Then the whole bowl went dark and I couldn't see a thing. My head hurt, my eye hurt and the lightning bolt came back so fierce this time I thought I would faint. I had to step back off the stool and regain my belongings. I looked at the technician and asked when it would be over. "Five more minutes," she replied. My thoughts raced and it seemed like five hours to finish. Thank heavens the lab is just a pinprick I thought. I went to the lab after that and waited for my turn, as my head felt like it was about to pop. The technician drew the vials of blood and I finally was on my way out of the clinic. The minute I got in the car I took three advil, that's the only way to stop the pain in my head. Now I had to wait again to see what the test results were. I prayed all the way back to the office it wouldn't be something serious. My hands shook on the steering wheel and I was frustrated not seeing cars coming up on my left side. Oh please dear lord, get me there safely!

Two more anxious days passed and I received a call from the doctor. My pituitary is fine and the thyroid is slightly over active. This meant there was no reason for sight loss. It was a relief to know this but what was causing the problem? The doctor tried to get me in to get an MRI immediately. This time I delayed this test. Bob was going to have surgery and it was necessary to make sure that went well. I needed to be at the hospital with him and the girls. I decided to wait a week for the MRI and try to move on from there with the problems at hand.

We decided to take our trip to Indianapolis for the races that weekend even though the surgery was scheduled for Oct 1st. Dana and Chris went with us for a weekend of fun before we knew the storm would hit our family. Our road trip to Indy was a fun six hours filled with laughter. We didn't get too lost trying to get to the Motel this time. Bob always maps out where we are going and somehow manages to memorize the way. He's always had a good memory recall, something I have admired about him. We settled in to our suite we shared and decided to go out for Dinner at Red Lobster. That's the first time we learned Chris doesn't like seafood. We apologized and he was fine with the meal. During dinner, Dana asked how to use the crab claw snappers without getting everyone messy at the table, we giggled while I pretended the light in the room was dim but with my three dimensional vision gone cracking that claw was very hard. I prayed silently she wouldn't notice that my left eye was closed so I could line it up properly. No one noticed my dilemma, what a relief! We went back to the hotel after dinner then Bob and I went off to the pool for a swim. Dana and Chris were tired and fell asleep watching TV in the room. Bob and I laughed and giggled together like children at the pool. Then we sat poolside and relaxed with a drink and talked of his surgery to come the following Monday.

The next morning we were up early and off to the racetrack. Time trials were to determine which driver would be on the pole for the race the next day. We walked around the track all afternoon, taking time to sit in certain spots to rest and watch. Formula one cars are loud and fast. Dana and Chris had never seen them in real life before. It was also a great weekend getting to know the man that Dana was so crazy about. The sun was hot and scorching. One of the places we sat to rest at I had to quietly ask Bob if we could move. The cars would come up quick on the left side of me and the peripheral vision was almost gone. I couldn't see them coming no matter how hard I strained my eyes. I kept getting lightning bolt headaches then finally when I started to feel sick from it I asked if we could move to another spot. As usual Bob understood and made an excuse for us to move to the corner we were at last year. Much better view and it stopped the headache.

Later in the day we went out to dinner at a steak house then back to the motel. We all went back down to the pool and laughed about the fun day. Suddenly Dana noticed the sunburn on Chris getting worse and the poor guy shook and shivered in the pool. Bob, Dana, and I noticed the devil like horns on Chris' head where his hat didn't cover his forehead. We all started to laugh and Chris didn't believe us until we got back to the room could see for himself. The sun and heat had gotten to us all and we quickly decided to get some sleep so we could tolerate another day in the hot sun at the races.

The races were so much fun that Sunday. We walked and looked at all of the souvenirs. I had to break down and buy a cap to protect my eyes. Sunglasses alone weren't enough. Bob found a cap for his team and Dana did too. After that we found our "corner" then sat and talked until the race started. After the cars got going there was no talking, the engines were much too loud. Bob's favorite driver won again and we battled the crowd to the parking lot to begin our trip back home. Dana and Chris quickly fell asleep and stayed that way most of the way home. They woke up for supper and fell back to sleep as soon as we were back in the car. Bob and I talked and teased the kids they still can't keep up with their parents. We dropped them off at their house and wished we didn't have another hour to drive. Aja and Ryan watched the dogs for us all weekend and we knew they needed to get out soon. Back at home we played with Angel and Winston for a while and then dragged ourselves off to bed. There is nothing like your own bed after a long weekend of sheer fun.

Bob went to work that Monday to keep his mind off of his back surgery and to be sure everything was in order while he took the month off for recovery. I stayed home to get things ready for him and do a little cleaning knowing he would need help. I took the whole week off to help Bob. That day my mother and Aunt Joyce came to visit after Joyce had stayed with my aunt Betty who has liver cancer. My Aunt Joyce thought she wouldn't see her sister again. My mother had gone to pick up Joyce so that she could take her to the airport in Chicago on Wednesday. Mom was going to England with my Aunt because she feared flying. From there my mother planned on going to my Aunt & Uncle's Country Inn in Wales. She was to spend some time in England and enjoy some time away. My mother planned on getting information about family history on my mother in-law's side of the family. We had been working on getting information about the Foley side of the family for many years.

It turned out to be a beautiful October day. We sat out on the back patio talking about days gone by with my mother and my Aunt Joyce. Joyce is my father's sister. She has the red hair my grandmother had and very English Irish personality to go with it. We talked and laughed about the days when I was a child and stayed in England with them. We reminisced about Uncle Lionel, her husband that passed two years ago and about my father who passed five years ago. My father was her younger brother. I didn't know how much he talked about my girls and me until Joyce filled me in. After all, I had the first grandchildren in the family and my father adored the girls. When my siblings and I were children my dad played and frolicked with us as if he were a child himself. Once we started to become teenagers and independent minds of our own he seemed broken hearted. It was true he never wanted us to grow up. I tried to understand and get that information out of my Aunt why she had only had one child; she didn't respond but evaded the question. She talked a lot of how hard it was for her to take care of my grandmother when she lived with her and how it broke her heart to quit teaching as early as she did. Apparently Joyce enjoyed children but did not go further in her personal life.

The conversation turned when my Mother asked how I was feeling. I know she was asking about my eyesight. I informed her the tests so far show I don't have problems with my pituitary gland or the thyroid gland. I didn't let her know about my fears. I tried so very hard to avoid the subject and my mother wouldn't let it go. My eyesight was getting worse, I had lost the peripheral vision in my left eye, if I tried to see through just that eye I couldn't, it went black. My headaches were getting worse, the bolts hit hard and I got extremely tired after them. I couldn't see three-dimensional anymore and had to concentrate on what I was doing and where I was walking. As hard as I tried I just couldn't see white on white and gray colors blended also. Bright vivid colors were easier for me. I loved it out in the sunshine, I could see. That morning I had been studying what could possibly be wrong, already I was hoping what I had read wasn't true.

I quickly turned the conversation to my husband having surgery the next day. I was so scared for him. It hurt very deeply inside of me to watch him suffer in such pain. After so many doctor visits we knew the surgery had to be done. His spine was affecting the muscles in his leg and numbness was abounding in that leg. Bob could no longer bend or help with anything at home. Mowing the lawns and taking care of any physical work was my duty. That was getting harder for me to do. I would lie and say I was ok. When people weren't looking I would stop and take a breather because my headaches were getting more intense.

When my brother came over that weekend with a load of wood he caught me stopping and I lied to him too, I said it was the stress of the upcoming surgery. He knew that I had gone to different doctors for the other tests, I hadn't told him about my eyesight. Partial stories worked and appeased relatives, and me; I didn't have to explain much at this point. My own husband didn't know I had been going through so much. I lay awake at night worried if was going to be here for him and his back problems. I worried about my girls, how would they ever accept something was wrong with their mother? Would I see them graduate college, would I see them get married or my future grandchildren?

Bob came home at his normal time that day. He asked about the visit with my mother and aunt. He was talking about everything but the surgery pending in the morning. For some reason his confidence was high. I kept on trying to make him talk about his feelings about the next day to come. Bob was not about to budge an inch. Both girls called about what time to meet us at the hospital. Bob's brother and sister and Mother called wishing him luck. We packed his bag for the next day, although Bob had it in his mind like the last surgery he could go home that same night. It was the part he hated most was not coming back home the same day. The whole evening was a busy flurry of the next day to come. Really that was good; it kept us both busy and not tearful. By the end of the night we were both very tired and had to go to bed early. We had to get up by four a.m. and had to be at the hospital by five a.m. Bob slept soundly; I lay there and listened to him breathe for a while before I could fall asleep. My mind kept on wondering, the surgery, with my fatigue wondered how I would help him, these days it was hard for me to stay awake past eight thirty at night. I just kept praying silently for help.

Bob's surgery morning came. We got up and I had a cup of coffee. I felt bad; Bob was not allowed any liquids. The hot coffee helped me come around after a sleepless night. Bob was as calm as could be and was looking forward to knowing the pain was about to leave him. He never mentioned what was going on with me. I think he knew but was afraid to admit it to himself. Today was the day to concentrate on getting him well. We chided about the new English country garden we put in that spring. We talked of recovery and how much better life will be then for both of us. Then we walked in to the hospital and checked in.

Bob asked for the room with a view, joking with the girls at the check in desk. It was still dark outside and the waiting room was quiet. We took a seat at the couch and I put my head on his shoulder. Bob put his arm around me and assured me he was going to be fine. The look in his eye gave me some confidence, but not enough to know just yet how it would be for him. I kept on praying silently for him, my eyes never shed a tear, not yet.

A little later a woman came from the long hallway and asked us to follow her. We were on the way to Bob's room. I watched intently as to where we were going. From here on in I didn't have Bob's guiding hand to show me the way. We arrived at the room and he was to get in to his hospital gown. Bob kept on joking about the beauty of the gown and how he was falling out the backside. I gave him a robe and smiled. Aja showed up then and she teased her father about how he was so cute in the gown. It felt good to have her there; she was helping me keep it together. She had a nice bouquet of carnations for her father. We teased and laughed as we always do. Dana as usual was running late. I tried to call her and she was in the parking ramp. Before Aja and I knew it the nurse was there ready to take Bob for surgery. Bob readily got on the gurney and kissed us both before he went down for surgery. I got teary eyed then and Aja put her arm around me. "Mom, Dad will be fine, you know that." I did know that, also I didn't quite know what was going on with me. I couldn't tell her, not yet. I wanted to, I wished I had someone in my family I could talk to about what was happening to me. This was not the time; I wanted the girls to think of their father and concentrate on how he was going through such a difficult process. Dana showed up then, she had a balloon and was her usual bubbly self. We fixed up Bob's room with the flowers we had and tried to not look where the bed was. I couldn't take it anymore and wanted to walk. Walk away the stress, walk myself through denial that I too was facing something major with my health.

It was an unusually warm October day. We walked the grounds of the hospital. We talked and the girls tried so hard to make me giggle. It was not an option for me today. I talked about how the day was so nice and warm and how the sun felt so good. Aja and Dana showed me where they went in and out of the campus near by. They talked about college and how I didn't get to go and how much they enjoy learning. I was so proud to hear that out of my adult children. They talked about their dad, I don't remember hearing much more than that. My mind raced about Bob. I worried if the nurses were taking good care of him; I worried about the anesthetist doing his job well, and the doctor, was he having difficulty and could he do what he promised. The anxiety overwhelmed me. Suddenly I just had to get back to the room where the empty bed was. I didn't hear what our girls were talking about there; I just wanted to know how my husband was doing.

We had gotten back to Bob's hospital room in time. He was in recovery and the surgery went well. Doctor found a spur that had grown in to the spine and rubbed on his sciatic nerve. He was able to remove it and fix the discs that he wanted. He made them in to a horseshoe shape, which would make them heal and relieve the pressure. Doctor was mostly excited about getting the spur out and being able to stop the numbness in his leg. If Bob had leg jumping it didn't work, if not he would regain the feeling in his leg. This was phenomenal. The prior surgery didn't cure this problem. It stopped Bob from losing feeling and falling, which was so dangerous, this find that didn't show up in the MRI's and it was so hopeful for Bob. Time would be our answer.

Finally they brought Bob back to his room. We three girls crowded around his bed. Waiting for him to see us and know we were there. He slept a little and finally I had to kiss him and let him know I was there. While we waited for him in surgery we went to the gift shop. The girls and I found a couple of things that we hoped would make him happy. Bob lay there silently; we waited in anticipation. Finally he opened his eyes. The weak smile told us he was doing fine so far. Dana & Aja said "Hi Daddy," I stepped back. The girls had to know Bob was still with us. They jabbered at him as usual, when I could see it annoyed him I gently prompted them away. Again, I leaned over the bed and kissed his forehead, and smiled. "I'm so glad you are back with me" was whispered; Bob smiled meekly, and replied, "I wouldn't be anywhere else." My eyes got teary, knowing he was fine. It was time for him to rest. I held his hand a minute and informed him we would go for another walk, he could nap and feel a little better when we returned. It was still unusually warm and the walk seemed like a good idea. October had not seen 80 degrees F. for years, we all felt over heated. The girls and I laughed about things in the past during the walk and discussed how long it could be before Bob would be up walking again. Anticipation would be early evening to get his circulation going again. We looked at the fancy cars in the parking lot that the doctors owned; we walked past the University again that was near and both girls showed me where they went to classes this time. Both girls had been and were going to that school for different courses. I was thankful they didn't notice how closely I was watching the ground and how the colors of the cement on the road seemed to blend and the obstacles in the way of my eyesight were affecting me. It was the feeling of a glaucoma patient or perhaps someone with a cataract. When I tried to close my right eye the sight in the left eye would go black, when I used both eyes it was like something was in my way, dirty glasses feeling. I kept thinking the lasik surgery went wrong, the flashes of light in the eye were from something done in my cornea or retina. I read that people cannot tell the whites against each other and that is exactly what I was doing. Dana said something about the races we had been to over the past weekend and started to say "right mom." I don't have a clue what she was talking about but was grateful she brought me back to the reality of taking care of Bob now and to try not to worry about myself. I was going to have an MRI done on Saturday and would try to stay focused. I lost concentration again and asked that we go sit with their father again. We went back to his room, Bob had just started to awaken from his nap and the nurse was checking his vitals. The blood pressure was good, and his heart rate was fine, although they were worried about the wheezing. The nurse was going to have a respiratory person come work with him. The nurse gave him a "clicker" in his drip so that when he felt he needed some pain reliever it would be right there for him. We were waiting for the doctor to come talk to us and check on Bob again. We watched junk day TV, and giggled about the people on the programs.

Finally the doctor came in and reported that Bob was doing well. The doctor went over the surgery again, so many details to remember and said he would check in again later. We had to wait for his approval and for Bob to be able to try walking again. The respiratory therapist came in and had him work on the breathing techniques. It was getting close to noon and it was quite apparent that Bob needed a nap. We girls were starting to feel a little hungry again, so it seemed a good time to go the cafeteria for a bite to eat and let Bob take his nap.

The room was full and they had lots of good food to offer. The doctors were at a table comparing notes from the morning. Bob's doctor was there also. He greeted us and assured us he was fine. I replied, "Doctor I know you did a good job, I can feel it. We have confidence in you." He is such a nice man as well as a known surgeon in our part of the country; I knew the fearful part was over. Now it was up to Bob to obey orders and work on recovery. The lunch line was quick and I can't even remember what we ate other than being women we treated ourselves to a completely fattening dessert. They gave us so much we couldn't finish. The girls and I discussed how glad we are everything went better than expected. We looked at the other people in the cafeteria, patients with their families, patients taking a break from dinner in bed and trying to walk so they can get out of the hospital and families obviously concerned about a loved one. The girls said they were so glad that is over, the worry about their father and how they were looking forward to helping him recover. The girls also discussed how they are happy they don't have to go through something like this again. I looked down at my half eaten cake and felt sick. I couldn't tell them, not yet, no more reports yet. I didn't want them to know I that was in pain from headaches, they took my breath away. I didn't want them to know we were working on me, and most of all, I couldn't tell them how afraid I was. No one but me knew, not the girls, not Bob, no one. I was terrified; was my sight going to leave me altogether? The man with the walking stick across the room was all I could see, the cane with red and white so we all knew he couldn't see. That choking feeling overcame me again, need to walk, even run overcame me again. I needed to get up and think of something new. I didn't want to break down; I didn't want to cry, not in front of the girls. With that feeling I jumped up from the table, grabbed my tray and said, "Let's go see if they will let us see the babies." Dana & Aja loved that idea.

We hitched a ride on the elevator and went up to the maternity ward. The lobby was locked and we could see people anticipating a new arrival or waiting to see the new baby. One woman brought her new prize package out. All we could see was the little blanket bundle and the pride from mom and dad's face. I stood there and reminisced with the girls about the day they were born. I laughed about how Aja was in a hurry from the start and how Dana took things slowly. Dana, our first-born took a whole weekend to come and see us, from that day forward she liked to absorb things around her. Aja's birth announced she was in a hurry and was not going to let anyone stand in her way. I looked at my watch and saw it was a little over an hour since we had let Bob sleep and how we should get back to the room to see how he was. He was still resting and doing well, so we three girls decided to go up the hall to watch TV and not disturb him. We were watching *Days of our Lives*, Aja's favorite soap opera. The three of us sat there and I kept watching the program. Dana and I asked Aja what was going on in the show so we could follow the story. We were filled in and could understand what was happening and who mattered in the story line.

Something, I can't remember what triggered Aja to start her usual explaining her reasons for Dana and I to quit smoking. I think it was the thought of the respiratory therapist working with her father. She explained to Dana she was young enough to stop any damage and explained to her how bad it was for her allergies. Dana said she understood completely how her sister felt. Then Aja started in on me. She explained how she worried my smoking would take her mother away from her too soon. I listened about how she felt, intently. Then when Aja said, "I want you to see your grandchildren." My eyes welled in tears that wouldn't stop. I tried swallowing; looking at other things but the feeling could not be chased away. The tears would not stop. I couldn't talk, couldn't move, I just froze. I kept on thinking, "If you only knew, and I can't tell you yet." I don't know what is happening to me! The fear became overwhelming. I noticed my hands were shaking, my legs felt weak and I was so glad I was sitting on the love seat. "Mom," Aja became alarmed, "don't cry. I'm so sorry, I didn't want to upset you, I only want you here with me." By then my throat hurt, literally choking in fear and pain. My mind raced, my very best friends, my daughters and I couldn't tell you, not yet. "Oh honey, I know what you are saying, I am so sorry for crying, I'm just tired and so relieved about your father." That is all I could meek out. The guilt for not telling them what was going on caught my heart too.

By that time Bob had been resting for two hours. We decided to go back up the hall and check on him.

He was awake. "I thought you left me," he quipped, he knew better. "Oh, we waited for you to rest and see us more clearly this time," I retorted back. He just smiled. I could see he was in pain as hard as he tried to hide it from us. Again, he deserved a kiss for trying so hard, and his forehead was so warm. Without trying to alarm anyone, I asked when his temperature was last taken. Of course he didn't know. I gave him some ice water. Bob sucked through that straw like it was the last drink he was going to take. He leaned back again and his eyes got brighter. We watched the news and he could actually comment on what they were talking about. Recovery was going well. The girls and I sat there and waited for Bob to talk to us, he did, off and on to let us know the improvement was gradually coming. The afternoon passed along while we sat waiting and hoping for a wonderful recovery. Finally after another nap while we were watching *Jeopardy* he answered a question. We girls turned and looked at him in amazement. Bob is and will be the smartest man I have ever known, he can hold information like no one I have ever met. His daughters have come to expect it; simply from pride a father can hold on to for his children. I never doubted how smart he is, it's the fact of when you have been married for many years you would think you would know someone's level of intelligence. I don't think Bob will ever let on what that level is to me much less the rest of the world.

It was time for another nap and for me to let all of the family members know the progress of Bob's condition. I called Bob's mom and sister and brother. They wanted to talk later to know the end of the day results. Of course I promised to call when I had gotten home and Bob would rest for the night. I called my mother, the girls called their boyfriends. I tried to not let the girls know the whole conversation with my mom. She knew some and was so comforting about the surgery and Bob doing well. She did say how important it was for me to carry on with my tests. "Mom, one at a time, I can't concentrate on so many subjects right now. Please, let me enjoy this moment, my husband is fine, he just has to walk again." That sounded so absurd to me. I wanted Bob to walk; I wanted him to be fine. I had to get back to the room. I so needed to be with him. The excuses came to release my mother from the phone and go back to my husband. No more questions about me, never in my life had I been the center of attention and I don't want to be now. My thoughts raced once again. Finally of not really listening I understood enough of the conversation and said to my mother, "Please, just go to England with Joyce, don't cancel the trip." I had to think about the other people in my life, not me. Mom needed to get away. She needed to connect with her family in England again; she had been lonely since Dad died.

I stood in the parking ramp looking at our girls. They were busy with talking to Chris and Ryan. They looked so relieved about their dad. I sort of listened to them and watched the smiles on their faces. Dana told Chris she was so happy her dad was fine. Aja told Ryan the same. It felt nice for that moment to see the smiles across their faces. As I watched them the thought chilled through my spine again. I can't tell you how afraid I am. The moment of knowing your father will be better again is so comforting to us. I hated feeling like I was lying to them. I wanted so badly to tell them I was hurting inside and didn't know what was going on with me. At that point I decided to enjoy the moment and know I had to let Bob heal. One obstacle was removed. My girls, as much as a mother I have been to them, they will never know how much I had depended on both of them. If any mother could feel anything this was the time. As I looked over at them I saw such beautiful people. Dana, the girl with knowledge that came easily, and it happened all of her life. I hoped and prayed for our daughter to have faith and confidence in herself. She had been a shy child, a person who felt she needed reassurance but really she had it inside of herself. She's a bright and patient person. A girl who has everything to offer to the right people, kindness, intelligence and such a silent beauty that it catches you off guard if you're not careful. Aja is our very forthright child. Life and opinions will be her way or no way. Our bright and beautiful second child. She is also what a parent dreams for when they think of a child, a person with sensitivity, intelligence and beauty that stand out. I watched our daughters with awe, and said a silent prayer. How lucky can Bob and I be? We have so much to be proud of with our daughters. My thoughts turned sour again. How am I going to handle what they tell me? How am I going to take care of my husband? I want to be there, for you Bob, for you Dana and Aja and I don't know. My head hurt again, my eyes hurt, the right eye from trying so hard to compensate for the left, the stress of the day, praying Bob was fine and the doctor could take care of him.

We went back to Bob's room hoping they would allow him to walk again. The evening was drawing near. I was fretting driving home in the rain and couldn't say a word. Dana, Aja and I were getting tired. We were excited Bob could eat his dinner without problems. He was getting more and more aware of his surroundings. Bob was asking questions about the day. His surgery and what the doctor had said. Bob was clarifying his mind. This too was a good sign. We watched the thunder clouds move in from his room. The day was nearing 7 p.m. It was such a long day, filled with worry and confusion, then relief. I sat in the recliner and rested while Aja kept running up the corridor to the nurse's station to get popsicles for her dad.

Dana watched him with worried eyes. She was definitely nervous and couldn't react to it. Aja worked her nervous feelings through with running for things for her dad. We giggled on how we spent part of the day at the gift shop trying to find the right thing for Bob. We told Bob how we walked and talked and hoped all day for him to do well. His beautiful blue eyes shone like a bright star. He wanted to get up and walk and try his new spine. We all knew how important that is for recovery. The nurse wanted him to wait a little longer.

Darkness and rain were getting closer. Lightning was striking out the window of the room. We could hear the rain hitting the window of the hospital room. My fatigue was beginning to overcome me. Dana had to get up at five in the morning. It was only eight by this time. She had an hour drive home. Bob asked her to go and assured her he was fine. She could tell and felt comfortable with that. She leaned over his bed and kissed him good night. Her daddy was fine and the nurses would make him walk. We agreed that it would be best for her to call me at 10 p.m. to see how he was. Aja watched me, she could tell without saying a word how I was feeling. "Mom," I want to stay, "you have over an hour drive home, plus when you get there you have to call the rest of the family. Please go home and rest. I will make sure dad walks tonight. My drive home is only 10 minutes. " I didn't want to leave. I made her promise to call me. I felt like I couldn't hold my head up anymore. I knew Aja would take care of her dad. How could I tell Bob, Dana or Aja the mere thought of driving in the rain frightened me? I knew my sight was so bad it would be hard to see. The lines mixed in to two, my vision at night was double. At that point I quietly tucked my left hand in the right to stop the trembling. Bob asked me to leave and call the family and him when I got home.

Somehow he knew, I never told him how I drove at night with one eye closed to avoid the double vision.

How did he know?

It was the worst drive ever. The rain enhanced my double vision.

The lines were two on the right and two on the left. My wipers were working just fine on the car. I wished they would take away that double vision. I concentrated and drove very slowly. I wrote down the directions to the hospital and home. In the rain I could see things popping out at me that weren't there. The road was dark and very lonely feeling. My eyes were teary from fear. I don't think I have ever driven with my hands so tight on the wheel before. The lines on the road kept on turning in to one. I closed my left eye and could see better. The rain poured down, harder and harder. I almost wished a patrolman were near, if I explained to him would he drive me home? If I told him I was afraid to drive would he understand? The country road I had to encounter was much worse. The two-lane highway turned in to four. I concentrated more than ever before. I closed my left eye, to decrease the double vision. My head hurt like never before. The "lightning bolts" of pain made me feel ill. Every bolt made me jump; every car that went by I prayed I would never hurt that person. My greed made me want to save myself. I want to make Bob better. I want me to get better. What am I going to face? My fear made me tremble again. At that point I made myself practice breathing slowly. In with a deep breath, exhale slowly. I saw my turn coming, finally. Drive up highway G, down Decorah and you're home. Rain kept hitting my windshield, I tried to see, oh God please, get me home!

I stepped in the back door. Home. Oh my goodness, that was the worst drive ever. I was actually panting and shaking. I stood there and composed myself. Angel and Winston were whining. How wonderful; something else to think about ran through my mind. It was such a relief to be in my kitchen. I let the dogs out of the gate and let them run through the back yard. They were confused about Bob not being there. I fed them and was grateful Ryan came up to the house during the day to let them out and play. He is so good with the dogs, it's as if they are his own.

The phone rang. It was Aja. Dad walked, she exclaimed. What a relief. Stood there with him and helped him. The tears welled up in my throat. I wasn't there. Instead I told no one how the drive home would be so bad for me. "Oh honey, I can't thank you enough," I replied. She asked if I had made any calls yet, I responded no. "Mom," Aja said," you should have been home 45 minutes ago." How do I cover this one? "How was the walk for Dad?" Her excitement was so great she forgot the long time it took for my drive home. Bob did well. He wasn't off balance, he joked around and the relief became overwhelming.

"Wonderful," I told her, "oh honey, you helped me more than you will ever know." The details of Bob's first walk after surgery made me so happy, he was going to be fine. The feeling came through me like a tidal wave, my husband made it. The pointed question came from the hospital room in the background, what took me so long to get home? Again, the total evasive reply came, "The weather was bad, and the rain and wind made me drive slow." I turned the question around again, "Please be extra careful on your drive home." Aja wanted to wait another hour until she knew her father was resting before leaving the hospital. She called Dana and filled her in on her father's progress. We all felt so much better. At that time I decided it was time to let the family know. I talked on the phone to Bob's brother, sister and mother until 11 pm.

My head hurt like never before. It was nice to let my mother-in-law know her son was fine. She made plans to come down over the weekend. She would arrive on Friday. My mind raced and it was most definitely time for her to come and be with her son. I hoped she would feel comfortable at our home.

The next morning I was to be at the hospital by nine. The night was so restless. I am not used to having Bob gone. We have been together in the same house every night for the past 26 years. I was excited to have my husband home with me again. I didn't care if I had to help him, I wanted to. I love him; to me it seemed the biggest honor a wife could do for her husband. It was time for me to get ready to go to the hospital and get him. I looked at the clock on our bedside table. It was only 5 a.m. Oh no, I have to try to sleep for another two hours. Angel and Winston slept with me. I listened to them snore. Wishing I could.

The green numbers on the clock were just fine with my right eye. I tried to stare and found the numbers disappeared. I closed my left eye. The numbers stayed where they belonged. I tried with both eyes; again the chill hit my spine. That time on the clock left my sight. It went black in the room when I tried to see out of my left eye. I concentrated on the green digital numbers; they didn't come back. I couldn't see them. I needed to see light. I turned on the bedroom light. Angel and Winston squinted at me. I was elated to see the dogs. My fear came back. What are they going to find? What will the doctors tell me? At that point I just stood there, looking at our dogs. I had been frozen and couldn't move. I can't ever say how long the stance stayed, I can only say I remember looking at our bed, the dogs and wishing my strength would be there to help Bob, trying to not be afraid of what might be coming my way and to be completely grateful that Bob was going to be on the mend now.

For too many years I watched the man I love in pain. His back hurt so badly some times that it even hurt to sit and rest it. Everything that he needs in our home is waist high or above. Some days it's hard for him to even put a dish in the dishwasher. He would wince when he bent over to put on shoes on learned to pick things up with his toes if he was barefoot that fell to the floor. Bob had gotten so good at relieving the pain in his back that he could actually control a sneeze and a cough. For years he would have to have me take care of the chores that were simply too painful for him. It's a good thing I enjoy mowing the lawns and shoveling snow when necessary. Through time I had to learn which chores I could assign him so he could help with daily life. Some days I could see he tried to hide the pain; little did he know without a word I could see in to those blue eyes and tell he was hurting. Too many days have been spent in our lives together with hoping he could wake up some day and not have pain in his back, and too many compensating because there was. It hurt me as much as it did him. I would close my eyes and wish that I had a magical power to erase the pain for him like the old television sitcom "Bewitched." A wiggle of the nose and what is wished for comes true. When years of pain overcome you, a little fantasy takes one away to a safer and friendlier place.

Finally 6:30 came and it was justifiable to get up and out of bed. Angel and Winston were ready to eat. Angel had been snuggling with me the whole night. I love the way you can just wrap your arms around her and she falls contentedly asleep. Winston never liked confinement, so he hangs out at the bottom of the bed. This time he knew I was feeling low and came up on the other side and rested his big head on my chest. I lay there petting our two dogs and started talking to them. Pets are the best listeners ever! I could see in the dusk they were looking at me with such interest, or so I wished. They really liked me talking softly to them.

Winston and Angel started to hit me with their paws telling me it was time to get up.

Angel & Winston ran downstairs and wanted to eat. Angel will not go outside without breakfast first. Winston runs out and paws at the door wanting to eat. I didn't want to give them much not knowing how long it would be until we got home again. I brewed myself a strong cup of coffee to perk up from no sleep and such a stressful day before. I sat quietly without the television in the kitchen on, didn't want to watch the morning news and sipped on my coffee. The train of thoughts about bringing Bob home today and worrying about his health and how to be so gentle was on the forefront on my mind. I watched Angel and Winston play and encouraged them to so that they would be ready to rest right after I had gotten Bob home. I would only be gone for 3 hours this morning.

While I was sitting at the kitchen table the phone rang. It was my friend from work, Diane. She was checking up on me and offering her help. Diane, oh how I appreciate your friendship. We would take walks together on breaks at work. How we walk that mile and laughed the whole way through was amazing to me. Neither one of us lost weight but we sure tried to keep healthy. It was so nice to have someone so dependable. We laughed, we cried, we consulted about our families and work. Diane goaded me to get checked on my sight. She even threatened to take me to the doctor. She would be so kind and gentle but so assertive in her ways. Diane could tell immediately when something bothered me. We never had to ask questions to get the information as to what bothered each of us; it just spilled out. Somehow she could feel what I was going through that morning. Diane let me ramble on about how I was feeling. Even as insecure as my feelings were she reassured me it was normal and I was coping like a trooper. I hung up the phone and wished I felt that way.

The shower felt so good. I stood there under the heat and absorbed it into my muscles. Standing there in the shower letting it rain on me. My muscles tingled from the heat trying to relax me. I thought about the day ahead, my questions for the doctor were in the process of trying to get the correct information on how to help Bob. I stood there in the heat trying to think of the things I should look out for and ask about. Soap got in my right eye and I was trying to rinse it out. When I thought it was over I looked through my left eye and couldn't find the green and white soap against the shower stall. I couldn't see it! I stood there frozen, the room went dark and I was feeling faint. Quickly I shut off the shower, grabbed a towel off the rack, wiped my face and found light again. Another lightning bolt headache came at that instant. I held the towel rack to steady myself. Oh my, my sight was getting worse by the day. I couldn't tell three-dimensional any more. I had to close my left eye to find the way to not trip. I wrapped myself in a towel and headed to the bedroom. The clock said 7:00 am. This was fantastic as I was running right on schedule.

It was still a nice October day. I dressed and found some clothes for Bob. He needed easy to get dressed in things that would not strain his incision and make him comfortable for the trip home. Time dragged until I had gotten to the hospital. Traffic was bad, lined up on highway 43 from an accident and people trying to get to the city for work plus a plethora of college students trying to get to class on time. The parking ramp was full, of course. Finding a close spot was impossible. I drove through twice and then someone magically pulled out so Bob wouldn't have to walk so far. I zipped into that spot before anyone could take my place. I think I ran through the lobby trying to get to Bob's room. The elevator wouldn't run fast enough and people seemed to be in my way. I wanted to get to him in the worst way.

As I entered Bob's room he and his doctor were discussing the procedure and the directions he should follow. I smiled at them both. Doctor Stoll smiled with me and said, " I know, you have your work cut out for you." I looked at my husband sitting there in the chair and asked if he was going to follow directions this time after surgery. Bob had a couple of more tests to endure before they could release him. I read the release papers and listened to the doctor as to what was to be done when we got home. Bob passed the walking tests, even made it up the stairs with the physical therapist. We were both so happy. He didn't feel any numbness in his leg anymore, and enjoyed the feeling. His eyes sparkled. It was time to let him go home to let him finish recuperating. While the nurses did their work on him, I went to the pharmacy. His prescription was ready. I went back upstairs all equipped to take him home. Such relief went through me. My husband was doing well. When I got back to his room he was ready to leave. He tried to grab our carry on case with wheels. I took it from his hand and held his arm. I was so proud of him. Such a recovery from surgery! That is my man, a fighter, and a determined man. We got off of the elevator and walked through the lobby. All the way through the halls and lobby he was talking and laughing; his usual self. I was elated he was doing so well. As we approached the end of the lobby he asked if I had gotten his pills. Guess the medicine was working and I reassured him the pills were in my purse. We walked slowly. A man came around the corner with a cane for the blind. We helped him to go in the right direction. Bob could feel the fear that overcame me. "Honey, you're next, we're going to find out what is wrong." I stopped and watched the blind man go forward and marveled how he could be so independent. Not realizing how quiet I had turned, Bob said, "I won't let you get that far." "We don't know that yet, how am I going to survive by feeling your face?" Please honey, let me enjoy how you're doing so well." He knew I wasn't ready to cope with what was coming.

Bob napped off and on in the car on the way home. He tried to instruct me on how to drive; as usual. I just looked over and smiled at him. "Close your eyes and nap honey, you have another half an hour before we get home." He snickered, "That's a good way to tell me to shut up." I didn't think that way at all. I was so happy to hear his voice, although it sounded tired. He fell off to sleep again. We got to the corner before our house and I said it was time to wake up. "Honey, I will get you to the back door, let the dogs out and help you inside." He obliged for once! Angel and Winston greeted me with joy, as they always do. I opened the patio door and let them out to run. I turned to let Bob in and helped to the kitchen table to sit and let the dogs in. They knew he was uncomfortable and were gentle with him. He let them calm down; I gave Bob some water and helped him up to bed. The girls would be coming in a couple of hours and I needed to let Bob have some quiet rest time. The dogs settled down quickly and the house went quiet.

It seemed the perfect time to set my alarm on the cell phone and catch a half hour nap for myself. Before I knew it the alarm rang and I was awake again. I crept upstairs and Bob was sleeping well. Angel and Winston sniffed him and left the bedroom with me.

The phone rang; Aja and Dana were on their way. I was so glad they were going to drive together. I felt so lonely since they moved out but was so glad they shared an apartment together and watched over each other. Bob called my name and I ran up the stairs. I had to stop suddenly at the top of the stairs and hold the rail. Another shooter headache came and I saw stars this time. Breathe deep, breathe deep, I silently told myself; you can do this I reminded myself. I opened the door and Bob wanted to know who was on the phone. I let him know the girls were on their way. He smiled and fell back to sleep.

When the girls got to the house they were bubbly and chatty as usual. Bob slept through the first hour they were here. Aja heard him stir upstairs and I went to see if he needed help. He came down to the kitchen and sat with us and talked about the day before with us. Bob giggled as much as he could and wanted to know how big the bandage was on his back. The gauze was about five inches by five inches. The phone rang again, my mother-in-law wanted to know the progress and how he was doing. Aja had class and Dana had to work so the girls only stayed a couple of hours. It was nice of them to come and see their Dad and that was just enough time for him to need to rest again. The rest of the day was quiet. I did some chores around the house to get ready for my mother-in-law to come for the weekend and tried to rest in between checking on Bob and feeling complete relief he was doing well.

After a good night's rest Bob was ready to get up and have some coffee and a small breakfast. My mother called in the morning to see how we were doing before she left for England with my aunt. Mom sounded like she was hoping I would ask her to stay home and I encouraged her to go. We won't know anything until the MRI had been completed and the doctors read the reports. Reluctantly she agreed to go.

She wanted to call me on the Sunday following my exam and I asked her to wait until the week after. No one will know the results until all of the tests are complete and it would seem foolish to try second-guessing the situation. I stressed to her this is my time to help Bob and relax with him. My focus was on him at this time. Finally I had gotten her to understand. It was so hard to not say how frightened I was. It was hard to not ask my mother to come hold my hand and tell me everything was going to be fine. I spoke with my Aunt Joyce for a while and was happy she felt content to go home and not be fearful she was going to lose her sister. I thought how my own sister didn't know a thing about what was happening to me. I swore my mother to secrecy, along with my brother.

Paul came by the next day and was worried about how I was. He scolded me for telling my mother the whole story as to what has happened so far. He had a hard time understanding my mother could hear in my voice there was something going on with me. I asked him to please let me handle this my way. He asked me to tell the girls. It wasn't time for that yet and finally he agreed with me. This is Bob's time now, he needs to heal and feel comfortable before I can take another step forward. I informed him Bob's mother would be here later in the day. Paul decided to be his usual busy self and would come back later to see Jennie.

Judy and Ken were on time as usual. They admitted Bob's mom didn't want to wait another minute to check on her son. We had just gotten back to the driveway from a little walk. Bob's family was surprised to see he was up and walking around the block. Everyone came in the house and relaxed for a few minutes and then Judy and Ken had to leave. They were working on painting their house and the weather was good and wanted to finish what they could before it turned cold again. I fixed lunch for the three of us and we chatted a while. Bob was getting tired and went back to bed for another nap. Bob's mother went to the couch in the family room and started to watch television. The dogs were cuddled in her lap and all three decided to take a nap. The kitchen needed to be cleaned up before I could do the same. As soon as I sat down to rest the phone calls started again from family members wanting to know how recovery was coming along for Bob. I gave the phone to his mother during each call so she could talk to them also.

That evening after supper the girls came by again and Paul came to see my mother-in-law. We laughed at the table about times past. Bob got up from another nap and came downstairs to join in on the conversation. He started talking about a program he was watching. I smirked at him, "Honey, we don't have a television in our room." He started to laugh about it and asked me to check his prescription for painkillers to make sure the dosage was right. It seemed to scare him. Bob's mother, Paul and the girls and I laughed. We sat and chatted some more and then it was time to call it a night. Paul wanted to get home and let his puppies out and then go to bed for a good night's sleep before he started another long day at his factory. We were all exhausted by that time and felt the same. The girls needed to get home too, they have long days with work and school. Bob's mom and I waited until he was asleep and went off to bed too.

Friday came quickly. Bob's mother decided she would take care of him and I should go to work. I agreed to go for half a day, that way I could check on clients and tend to some work that needed doing.

Diane was surprised to see me there. Obviously Bob was doing well enough that I felt I could leave. There were a lot of calls to take care of and lots of questions to answer from co-workers. It was nice to hear how they cared. Diane made me go for the morning walk and relieve tension. She let me chatter on and on, at the same time reassured me about the tests I was going to take on Saturday. Just hearing her voice and letting me know I was doing well with the situation made me feel so much better. After break I called and checked on Bob and his mother. They let me know the things they wanted at the store on my way home. When I arrived home I found a box of goodies Bob's boss had sent to him. He and his mom had a good time with the treats in the box. They both were ready for lunch even though they had snacks. I teased my mother-in-law about not feeding my husband with healthy food. "Oh no," she said, "that's your job." She chuckled. I made us all lunch and by then Bob was relieved I was home so he could nap again. Bob felt he needed to entertain his mother. He went up to bed and slept soundly. Bob's mom went back to the family and started to watch television. After dishes were cleared and Angel and Winston went out I went to join her. The two dogs quickly invited themselves to her lap. She sat there and petted those wonderful soft ears they have. I checked she was comfortable the night before in the bedroom she slept in and she said she hadn't slept that well in months. I don't know if she was just saying that but left it that way in hopes she was comfortable. As we were talking about Bob and other things she nodded off to sleep with the dogs in her lap. I watched television for a while and she woke up after I had gotten up and checked on Bob. I giggled when I got back downstairs to see her sleeping. I felt bad because this woman had been so busy at one time in her life and now the years had caught up to her. She woke up and said she was sorry. I explained with the cozy puppies in your lap it is so easy to drift off and it happened to me all the time

The rest of the evening went calm and smooth. Bob got up for a while and talked with his mother. It was so nice to see the two of them together. I sat there listening to all of the things that made them happy during years gone by. I even felt envy. My family wasn't that way. They said bad things about each other. We talked about Dad Saler and how he would have been right there walking with Bob. We all miss him and wish we could spend just one more night with him. The girls called. Dana had taken vacation time off for the next week to come stay with her father. She wanted to talk to Bob and her grandma. Because of her job she couldn't come up until the evening the next day. Aja was busy with her job and full time school. She needed to work and go to school until late that day. She talked to her grandma for a while and her father to be sure he was doing well. Both girls were looking forward to the visit the next day.

Saturday morning came quickly. I had to lie and tell my mother-in-law I had an appointment with a customer who needed house insurance. Bob knew I was headed off to the clinic for an MRI. He reassured me they don't hurt and that I would just hear a lot of banging noises. My appointment was at 9 am. I drove there in guilt about not telling the family and wishing I had Bob to help me. Saturday traffic is light that time of day so I made it there quickly. I checked in at the desk and sat in the waiting room feeling very anxious. It seemed like hours and it was only ten minutes before the lab technician came to get me. I had to take off all of my jewelry. As I was taking off my necklace, earrings and rings she explained the procedure and how they were going to inject a dye in me at the end of the MRI. As she gave me the earplugs I recalled Bob telling me about his past experiences and felt comforted reliving what he had told me.

They strapped me on a hard cold table. The technicians put a small pillow under my knees. As one of them was talking to me she began to put a restraint on my head. "You cannot move your head while we are taking pictures" and began to tell me how the MRI machine worked. I sort of heard her. I wanted to get up and run. "If you sneeze this will hold your head still." She gave me some earplugs and I know I looked confused. "You will hear loud banging noises." This is going to protect your ears. Are your comfortable?"

"Um, no," I replied, "I'm about to go in a big machine that shoots radiation and pictures of my head and your standing on my left side where I can't see you but can hear you and I am terrified what you and the doctors are going to find. If you're asking if I am comfortable lying here yes, I haven't had a chance to relax like this in days." She went on with the medical descriptions of what was going to happen. I lay there hoping there would be an answer and also afraid of the answer that was going to come my way. The machine started to suck me inside, or so it felt that way. I heard very loud banging noises. I heard another machine making a noise like the wind was blowing through. I heard David Bowie singing Space Odyssey; I heard the alarm system telling me this is a test, only a test. If I there had been an actual emergency we would have been told where to tune in and where to get safety. I blinked thinking these thoughts were silly.

The machine kept on making banging noises like it was going to blow up. I lay there hoping it wouldn't.

The technician came up next to me as the hard cold bed moved me out of the machine. She injected a dye into my arm and said I only had ten more minutes to go. I was sent back into the machine and listened to more banging. The technician pulled me back out and helped me sit up. I felt dizzy and wanted to sit a minute. Suddenly my headache came on again, I knew it was happening all over. "You are now a little radioactive from the injection but not dangerous to anyone." I looked at her strangely. My thoughts raced and listened intently how in the next 24 hours it would be gone. "Doctor Boyd will call you with the results." "It will take two or three days." I thanked them and was given my locker key for my purse and personal belongings. After I had dressed I headed out of the clinic. When I had gotten to the car I had a bottle of water and took some Advil. Headaches please go away, I have to drive and take care of Bob. I sat in the parking lot a minute and gathered strength to make it home.

The drive home was filled with wonder. What will they find? Am I in serious condition? My sight, is it a quick fix like everything else in my life had been? I wanted so hard to concentrate on the road and my hands just kept on shaking on the wheel. I held the wheel of my Volkswagen Jetta and thought of how proud I had become of owning this car. I looked at the black interior and the fixtures on the dash and marveled how much I enjoyed driving this car. Anything to stop myself from wondering the thoughts that would destroy what I was trying to do; find out what was going on with me and trying to concentrate on my husband who was recovering from back surgery. I had to make it home to take care of him; I had to pretend that nothing was wrong to my family. How do I find out what I have to do and take care of my family? I looked up at the road ahead of me, knowing my mother-in-law was staying at our house I decided to try to calm my nerves with a cigarette. My mother-in-law hated me smoking and has no idea her son does, to respect her we don't smoke in front of her.

When I had gotten home Bob was outside. His mom didn't make it as far as he could walk. He was standing there waiting for me to come home. I asked where Mom was and he replied, "She's inside, I took her for a walk and she wanted to sit down." "Is she Ok?" I asked. He said, "Oh sure, she is just getting on and a lot of exercise is hard for her:" I looked at him and smiled. It is so hard to watch the people that helped us through life to become tired. "Your mom is now 86, it's a miracle she can do what she does," I said in a meek way to Bob. Let's walk a little more; he wanted to keep going. It felt so nice that he wanted to keep walking and it felt good on his back. I couldn't help myself but look at him and smile. Bob looked down at me and asked what I was thinking. "Honey, it is so nice to see you doing so well, your color is good, your feet are in line again and you're not complaining of pain," I said. He looked at me with all seriousness on his face, "It's been a little while now and you have not said anything about what you went through this morning." I tried to joke about it. "It's like being in a big tube with loud noises that hurt your ears and make you feel just like the old movies where we imagined space technology curing us." I continued, "You remember those old things on TV that used to say 'this is a test' and when the noise begins you can hear David Bowie singing Ground Control to Major Tom." Bob stopped walking and turned to me. "Yes, I remember well, that wasn't the song I heard in my head, but it sounds like your frame of mind." We kept walking a bit more and I was concerned he was overdoing it. "Are you ok?" He just felt so good about getting around without pain. It felt so nice to see him not wince and want to keep going. "Hey honey, let's head back to the house," I retorted, "we don't need to leave your mom alone for long." It was an excuse to make him slow down a little. Bob stopped me and turned around. His deep blue eyes caught me off guard again, he held both of my hands, looked in to my eyes with fear, "Cheryl, we are going to get through this, we are going to find out what is happening to you, I am not going to let you hurt." Oh my, my mind raced, he loves me so much and doesn't want me to hurt, and I could see it. I don't want to hurt you either I was thinking silently. I am so sorry, raced through my mind, I hate this, I hate feeling this afraid, and I hate feeling like I am hurting you, I hate hiding from our family and most of all, I hate thinking and knowing I am keeping this from the girls. I am their mother, the rock in their lives. I am your wife, the rock in your world. I have been there for you in everything you wanted to explore and supported you. I thought about the girls, I promised them I would be there for them. Is it going to be cut short? Do I get the pleasure of seeing them graduate college; am I going to see marriage and grandchildren? I couldn't tell Bob what I was feeling. Oddly enough I didn't have to. He grabbed me and held me when we got to our driveway. "We will get through this honey," and he held me tight.

We walked in to the house and found Mom sitting at the table. "Did the kids behave for you?" Mom Saler was ready to rest. "How about a little lunch?" I asked. I made some soup and Bob was ready to rest again too. Mom went to the family room and the two dogs cuddled up to her.. It was so peaceful to watch them. I made sure Bob was comfortable in bed and he fell asleep right away. I sat on the couch and watched the dogs and my mother-in-law drift off. I was about to do the same and had to capture the phone before it woke anyone up. My sister-in-law was on the phone. They were making progress in painting and wanted to pick up Mom the next day. That was fine with me, let her rest and spend time with her son.

Sunday morning came in its usual fashion. I was feeling tired again and couldn't say anything. Bob and his mother got up after me and I proceeded to make a brunch. Judy and Ken would be here around noon to get mom. Bob's mother enjoyed the feast I made for her. She even liked the turkey bacon. We explained to her how we didn't eat the hard fats anymore in real bacon. It was nice for her to come enjoy and see how her son was living. It seemed to make her happy that he is comfortable. I hoped I was fulfilling her wishes as a daughter-in-law, that I can make her son happy and feel fulfilled with his life with me. I hoped she could sense that I loved her son and would give the world to him if possible.

Judy and Ken showed up by 11:30 wanting to get on with finishing their house. I looked at my sister-in-law knowing I would have to give her another burden. I saw a woman who conquered cancer and wondered how she felt about the whole thing. She never talked to me about it. I wanted to understand and wanted to tell her what I thought

I was facing. Judy, so strong and so forthright; what made her that way? I envied her courage; I envied how she kept it a secret. I looked at her with amazement. If I tell you what they suspect will you reject me? Will you understand? I can't tell you anything; I have to find out what is going on, I have to let my girls know after Bob. Can I do this?

Monday morning the workweek was to begin again. Dana had the day off to come watch her dad. I went to work pretending nothing was wrong. I worked on pending policies, training a new hire and trying to make sales and earn commission. Diane and I walked on our breaks. She asked all about the weekend and how my tests went. I couldn't give her an answer yet. Diane let me speak about my fears, and aspirations. I have to wait, Bob has to continue to heal. My mind was racing. In the afternoon Amy came to work. She joined us and was trying to find out what was happening. I tried not to repeat myself but she wanted to know the progress. Every occasion that I had I would go to the teasing of her pregnancy. How she was eating crackers and looked so pale. How she was holding the baby. Amy was determined she was losing weight carrying the baby. I agreed. I wanted so much to think of something different and Amy turned in to the perfect person. She was having a difficult pregnancy and felt horrible. Encouraging her was easier than trying to do the same for myself.

I went home at my normal time that day after several checks on how the progress was going for Bob. Dana had prepared dinner for us and left shortly before I got home. Bob was relaxing and feeling better by the day. He and Dana watched and laughed at day TV. He gave me the run down on the day's events and was getting tired and needed to take a rest after dinner. I felt the same. I filled him in on my day at work and he listened intently. It was getting to the point where he needed more mental stimulation. Dana made him laugh and walked with him during the day. He was bonding with her again and it was nice to see. Those two have the same type personalities; they can clash and laugh at the same things at any given moment. Dana was happy with her new boyfriend and the glitter in her eyes told us so.

The next morning came in the usual way. A normal day to get ready to go to work and Bob was up and ready for Dana to come later. He enjoyed his time alone with the dogs but we were all fearful they would jump on him. Dana came up to our house mid morning to take care of her dad. They walked some more to help the healing process of Bob's back. The weather was still unusually warm for October. Dana decided to walk the dogs that day, she took Winston and Bob had Angel. I called home from work several times during the day to check on them and to see if I had gotten any calls from the doctor yet. I never thought the call would come that day because the radiologist needed to read the report. I would concentrate so hard on seeing out of my right eye, the left eye had become hopeless by this time. I looked at my paperwork on my desk and tried hard to concentrate on that. A customer called and broke my train of thought. It felt good to think of something else for a while. Diane and I took another walk in the afternoon and talked of what I was feeling. I kept repeating to her how I was praying there wasn't anything serious. All of a sudden I had to stop, my heart was racing and I felt dizzy. I grabbed Diane's arm to steady myself. "Diane, I am so sorry, guess things are catching up to me now." She just stood there looking at me for a minute and in her usual way replied, "Oh, I am so glad, I thought you were having a heart attack on me." I smiled at her little quip and tried not to let her see my eyes had teamed up with a tear. As usual she saw right through me. "You're going to be all right, you have to be." I kept on trying to ask questions about Tom and how the grandchildren were, and she wouldn't have it. "Cheryl, listen to me, you're going to be fine." As I looked I could see she too had weepy eyes. My friend was afraid for me. I started to feel so guilty for exposing her to this, my pain, worry and concern.

We walked back in to the office with our usual giggle stint. We tried especially hard at that time to not let anyone know at work what was happening. I respected Diane for letting me have my privacy. There were a few calls for me to return and I felt relieved to have to talk to others about their policies and rates. The rest of the afternoon went calmly and I was enjoying the feeling. I called home to check on Bob, he was resting and watching TV. He sounded relaxed and was going to try to nap before I had gotten home. Dana left a little early and needed to get things done at her place. She could tell by this time her dad wanted to be left alone. Again she had gotten dinner ready for me to heat when I had gotten home. She baked cookies and some extra to take home for Chris to enjoy. Dana is the queen of chocolate cookies, and still is. When I got home I put dinner in the micro to heat and had a cookie for dessert. After Bob and I sat quietly and watched the evening programs we enjoyed. It was nice to sit and daydream for a while. Not think of him healing, not think of wondering what was wrong with me. Time will give us the answers we are searching for and nothing can change this fact.

2.
Diagnosis

October 9, 2002:

Bob had an appointment with his doctor at 9:45 in the morning. A postoperative check and to get his staples removed. Doctor said he was doing well and removed the staples. He recommended Bob stay home from work for the next 5 weeks to finish healing. Bob rolled his eyes. I giggled and said it would be hard to keep him from staying out of work. His doctor explained again what was done for him and suggested to Bob he keep up with his walks and he was doing well with recovery. After he finished healing some more he would like Bob to take on some physical therapy to help the back muscles heal. With that we were both very happy.

We drove home along the freeway home and Bob was so happy he was allowed to drive again. It's so hard when you aren't allowed to drive. He has always hated it when I would drive and nit-picked me to death when I drove. It was a relief to have him drive this time. I couldn't tell him the sun was piercing pain in my head. The headaches were getting worse and the lightning bolt pains were becoming more intense. I kept hoping this would just go away. Suddenly a bolt came so fierce it made me gasp for air. Bob said, "What? I can see where I am going, I am driving just fine." I nodded and finally my breath came back. " I know you're just fine." He didn't ask another question and I was relieved to not have to explain. I was so concerned about bringing him down on his happy day. I just wanted to enjoy this day too, life with knowing he would be fine and appreciate we have accomplished another obstacle in our life together.

We left the car in the driveway because I had to go back to work. Bob wanted to be alone for the remainder of the day. Dana decided it was a good time to get some of her errands and chores done. Both girls called to see how the doctor appointment went for their dad and we were delighted to tell them everything was going well and the recuperation time was on schedule. They were so glad to hear their father had made it this far. We chatted with the girls for a while and then ate a light lunch before I headed off to work. As I was talking to them I would try to see out of my left eye, Bob crept up on me and startled me from the that side. I turned my head and smiled at him, trying to push back my worries.

I got in to work just as the bell chimed one. Oh good, I could just jump right in and think of something else for a change. I checked up on all the messages, called my clients and started in on the tasks that needed taking care of. A few minutes later, Donna, the receptionist rang my extension. "Cheryl, your doctor is on line two." My hands suddenly started to tremble. It was a good day so far, Bob was going to heal, and the thought of something else wrong terrified me. I looked at the phone on my desk for a minute. I spent time telling myself everything was going to be fine. I didn't want to pick up the phone. I sat there looking at the buttons and thought it can't be put off any longer. I wanted to know what was wrong with me; I wanted to get the strength to go forward with the unknown. At that point I took a deep breath and pretended not to be afraid and not let the doctor know how frightened I had been feeling.

"This is Cheryl," as if he didn't know who was on the phone. "Hi Cheryl," this is Dr. Boyd. "How are you feeling, is Bob's healing coming along well?" "Yes he is well, and yes I still am getting a lot of headaches, and yes doctor I am getting more lightning bolt headaches every day. I am getting very nervous about this call, I can feel you are going to tell me something I don't want to hear." My doctor paused, "Your perceptive and I really hate this phone call. These are the days I don't like being a doctor. Are you sitting down? He didn't pause anymore. You have a menengioma. It's a tumor on your brain." The doctor took a breath like he was hoping I would understand. "What are you talking about? Can you explain this to me?" He began, "A menengioma is a tumor that invades your meningies on the lining of the brain. Yours has grown to be quite sizable and I would like to have you see a Neurosurgeon this coming Friday. I have already arranged the appointment for you at 10 am. You will go to the medical college hospital." The shock hit me. "Doctor, I am not understanding you. I have never heard of this before. Telling someone they have a brain tumor is like telling them you have cancer or heart disease." "Yes," he replied, "it is. You need to pickup the images before you go for your appointment." "Right, you are telling me I have a brain tumor, you don't know what the mass is and you want me to see another doctor immediately," I replied. "Exactly, the films will be ready for you to pick up tomorrow." "Oh, please explain this again, I am so off guard by this I need to hear it again." He did just that and said he will read all of the reports the doctors have and would be there for Bob or me for any questions. I sat there in complete shock. I don't know how long, I just stared blankly. My desk became a blur, the papers blended. It felt like a bad dream.

I put the receiver down. I sat and looked at it for a few seconds. The shock was overwhelming. I decided to pick up the phone and try to reach Bob. It rang and rang then the answering machine picked up. My mind was racing. I can't leave a message; I can't just call him and tell him over the phone. I threw the receiver and it bounced off of my desk. I tried silently to get the receiver from the other side of the desk. When I put it back on the receptacle the phone seemed like my enemy. The fear overwhelmed me and I just sat there and cried. My receptionist asked her assistant to answer the calls. She came in to my office and just hugged me. "Donna, I have a brain tumor" when I looked up at her.

"The doctors can't tell me anything more. I don't understand this. I can't see very well, my head hurts." She held me tighter, "You are going to be fine, and it's a hurdle." I looked at her with disbelief.

Shortly Diane showed up in my office. I don't know who summoned her. I can't even remember how I went in to my boss' office and told him I have to leave. He sent Diane out with me to make sure I could drive home. I told Diane what I had just learned. She stood there in shock and couldn't say anything. I explained what I knew so far. My body hadn't shook that hard since it was time to give birth to my daughters. I could hardly speak; I could feel a bolt headache coming on. I just stood there and cried. Diane in her so sweet way just put her arms around me. "Cheryl, I am praying for you. What can I do? Do you need a ride home?" When I looked at Diane in the eyes she went blurry. I blinked and chocked, "I have to go home, how do I tell my husband this? How will I tell the girls? I have to go, I can't stand here any longer." She argued with me about driving home alone. "I promise to call you when I get there." That was my very first time I really felt sorrow for hurting my friend. I had never done that before. I wanted to erase her pain; I hated the look of worry and the tears in her eyes. This was a new feeling for me. We looked at each other with such a stern honesty. "Diane, I need to drive my Jetta and feel free for a few minutes. I need to work on courage to tell Bob. By the time I get home he will be back from his walk and I can gather strength to tell him." Diane wanted to drive me; she had permission from our boss to try to get me home safely. "You are so nice to me, one day I will try to repay you." Diane retorted at me, "You have in so many ways already, I am trying to give back what you have given to me." I hugged her again and we held each other tight. "Diane, I am going to need you, can you help me? I need someone to bounce off what is happening to me, I need to talk to someone who will listen to my fears because I have so many right now. Would you please help me?" She smiled through her tears, "Of course, I am here for you." I looked into her eyes knowing what I was asking and wondered if she knew what was ahead. "I have to go home and talk to Bob, he is the most important person who needs to know at this time, and then I have to find a way to tell my girls." "Call me, let me know you are safe." I promised her I would and got into my car.

I sat there a second and looked at the key. A huge sigh came over me. Right, I can drive, I thought to myself. I watched the country road I had to travel and began to shake again. The barns that I passed daily became an obsession. I watched for my Shetland pony, he was outside, I watched for the veal farm even though it disgusted me to know they did that to calves. I looked at my brother's old farm and wished he were still there to stop and talk to him. The drive home I managed to stay dry eyed. The same route I took every day listening to music on my car stereo became different. The geographical markers for my time to arrive home became things that meant more.

Finally I arrived at our driveway. I pulled my car in to the garage and went in the house. Bob was still out walking to regain strength in his back. The relief came over me. I don't have to face him right away. I can sit here at the kitchen table and gathered some more strength to try let him know what is happening. I just sat with the dogs and petted them. I talked to Angel and Winston and shook again. Angel sat with her big sad dog eyes as if to say she knew. Winston did the same. I practiced my speech with them and did all that was possible to regain some courage. "Angel, Winston, how do I tell my husband I am so ill when all I have is headaches and can't see so well out of my left eye, how do I finally own up to what I have been going through without him being angry with me? How do I tell him, the man I love the most in my life that I could not live through this?" I sat there and pondered over the whole situation. My mind just reeled with the new information and trying to find a way to tell Bob first that I love him and then let him know that I will need him to help me. How do you tell a husband that you know loves you as much as you do him that you are this deep in health trouble? I had been there for all of his back problems and supported him. I had been there for all of his dreams and hopes for a better life. We shared all of this together for 26 years. Our children, our times of trouble: our times of happiness. We did this together, for the past 26 years. We went on a wonderful vacation to Mexico and celebrated 25 years of marriage. We are a bonded couple who share everything. Until recently, I was not truthful; I didn't want him to know how badly I was feeling. I ached with sorrow for not sharing this with him. I ached because I wanted to spare his feelings. It could not be hidden anymore.

Bob came in the back door, he was smiling. "I made over a mile on my walk. It's such a beautiful fall day!" My back didn't hurt for the whole walk. He was so excited he was feeling better. I looked at him, oh no I am about to burst your bubble of happiness is all I could think of. Suddenly he looked at me with a completely serious look. "You didn't come home to check up on me did you?" I just froze, my thoughts, my entire body. "No honey, please tell me more about the walk and your back; can we go out to the front room?" We sat in our respective chairs. Bob talked about how nice his walk was and how he was feeling so much better. I was so happy to hear his news. I listened so intently. Suddenly I was so thirsty and offered a drink for Bob too. He found he was thirsty and I had gotten a drink for both of us. When I returned to the front room with his ice tea and my ice water he confronted me.

"Cheryl, you don't leave work and you know I am healing at the pace the doctors want. You are hiding something from me, I know how you behave." I hung my head in shame. "Please, don't be angry with me. Please understand I wanted you to get healed for the most part before I went on with the tests. I wasn't honest with you about what was happening to me. I am so sorry. I was trying to protect us all." Bob grabbed my hand, "Tell me, what happened, I can take it, I can help you this time." I tried so hard not to cry and it wouldn't stop. "Honey," I sobbed, "I am very scared, I don't know the outcome of this, I don't know what the doctors want, I want you to hold me." He grabbed me and held me tight; I loved that feeling of security for that instant. "I'm so sorry, I want to be here for everything, the girls future marriages, Aja graduating college, she's only six months away. There are so many things I want to do. I want to be a grandparent with you, I want to enjoy life like we did before children, I want to be with you! I want to be old, together, I want to see my hair gray, I want to see, I want so many things that may be just taken away. How do I tell you I have a brain tumor?" The ramble just came out. I tried so hard to not spill it out that way. My body was shaking again; it trembled all the way through from my toes to my head. He held me closer, to the point to feeling like I was going to choke. I felt his pain; he tried not to cry in front of me. He just held me; he didn't say a word for an eternity in my mind. I regretted having to tell him this. I felt so bad for hurting him. It just didn't matter anymore what I was to endure, I hated hurting my Bob, he is so good and kind to me, he is my husband, this is the person I have tried for over 25 years to show my respect and most importantly the love of my life.

Bob put me at arm's length and looked at me squarely in the eyes. In my tears I could see his concern. "Honey, in all of that confession you just told me you have a brain tumor. How serious is this? What do you know? How long have you felt like this? Why didn't I push you to get more tests?" "Oh Bob," I tried so hard to explain, " I didn't know the tests would show this, I didn't want to hurt you." He just grabbed me again. "You were trying to tell me, I wasn't listening. I am so sorry." "How could I know? I wasn't honest with what was happening. I wanted you to get through the back surgery." Now it was time to fill him in what the doctor told me. I wanted to get all of the facts straight. It seemed like an eternity to tell Bob what was going on. " You can drive again, I need you to go get the MRI films and we have to go see a Neurosurgeon on Friday." We will know what to do from there. In the mean time it would seem to be a time to try not to panic."

We sat in silence on the couch just holding each other. Both of our minds were wondering. I looked at him with dry eyes this time. Bob just held me closer again. I could see he was in deep thought. He just smiled down at me; he kissed my forehead. I hated this feeling; usually I know what to say to make things better. My silence was finally broken. "Ok, where do we go from here?" Bob asked. "Well, we need to pick up a copy of the scans for the doctor on Friday. He will advise us from there. He will explain the MRI scans, he will let us know what to expect from here on in." I paused, it's only one day away. It seemed urgent to get in according to Dr. Boyd; he wants us to go for a consult visit. "Please come with me. I cannot do this alone. Bob's kind eyes reached mine for the first time through all of this, "I will not let you go through this alone, we will do this together."

Early the next day I had gotten up for work. "Where are you going?" Bob asked. "I have to try to keep on living, I may not get the chance anymore. I want to fight this." "Honey," he asked, "how long did you stay awake thinking about this?" "All night," I responded. "I have to live, I have to keep trying, and I just can't give up at this point." Bob was so understanding, he got up and gave me a hug. "I am standing right here for you. Lean honey, just lean on me, please. You are not alone. I am going to be here for you and we will together make the girls be strong for this one too. If you had not been here for me and for the girls we would be lost. Let us help you this time." I choked back tears. "Ok, I will warn you, I will go a little crazy, I will be hyper, I am going to cry, I am going to shake. Are you ready for this roller coaster?" He stopped for a minute, "I am going to ride with you this time." At that point I continued to get ready for work. As I was slipping into my skirt I tried to be casual, "Will you please go get the scans today? We need them for the appointment tomorrow." "Not a problem honey, it will be good to go for a drive." I left the bedroom full of thoughts. Bob promised to call with any information he had found.

On my way out the door I looked behind at my kitchen. We worked so hard to redecorate it the year before. I loved the way it looked. I looked down at Angel waiting for her pet good-bye for the day. Her little stubby tail wagged at me and I picked up her nose for a kiss. Winston came up behind her and I gave him a little kiss on the nose too. I grabbed my lunch box looking at our two dogs and wanted to stay home and cry but instead took a deep breath and headed out the door. For a minute I sat in my car and looked at the dials on the dashboard. When I started the car and buckled my seat belt a lightning bolt headache hit me again and the obstacles distorted my vision and the dials seemed to be half there. The shivers went up my spine and I couldn't move. Suddenly a happy song came on the radio and it calmed my nerves. I backed out of the driveway, closed the garage door and went off to work.

On the way I watched my familiar scenery. The farm with the veal cages I hated. I never ate veal just because of how those poor cows are kept. I looked at the poor things and wondered if they know what they are up against. I hoped they were comfortable. I hoped they didn't understand what was happening to them. A little further up the road was my brother's old farm. I hoped he was happy there. I hoped he would be happy in the road to follow him. I thought about how Angel lived there and she was given to us. My little couch potato puppy, who the first time I saw her on the farm she was sitting on a couch in the barn and how badly I felt such a cute dog just wanted a lap to sit in. She is such a proud girl, so pretty and so proper in her manner. I remembered the night how Paul had us come over to the farm and was primping us to take her home with us. A smile crept across my face and I remembered when we took her home to the family and she was so happy to sleep in a warm bed with Aja and be spoiled like she felt she deserved. Aja was so thrilled she came home with us, we even said "Happy Birthday," here is the puppy you wanted. The very next day Aja went out and bought all the puppy things she thought would make Angel happy. Angel was most happy with all of the love and affection Aja was giving to her. Dana went shopping with Aja too; between the two girls that dog was fit for a fine life with our family. Dana was mostly concerned about Otis. She spent her time making sure he didn't feel "replaced." It worked out perfectly, Dana adored and loved Otis to pieces and spread her attention to Angel when he slept. Aja did the same, and Angel sure didn't waste any time getting into the good graces of our family.

Further along the road was my little pond with the heron. He was so proud and staunch. He seemed to have lost his mate during the winter. I looked at the pretty gray blue color he was and hoped he didn't feel lonely. I always slowed down at the point of my travel to work to watch my heron for an extra second. He gracefully took a drink and he looked at my car as if to say "Hello." I nodded at him and wished he could be my friend to let me talk to him and tell him all about my fears. A little further along the way were the two horses that eat their breakfast when I am on the way to work. The Shetland was nibbling eagerly while her counterpart Palomino would look up after each bite. The big horse was wearing her coat again; I remembered how when I was a child my Aunt had a horse that had to wear a coat because he had such a bad case of saddle sore. I hoped that wasn't happening to that horse.

The final drive seemed to take forever. I thought about facing Diane and Donna and would keep taking deep breaths so that I wouldn't cry. I knew once I walked into work they would be full of questions. After I parked my car I tried to walk into work the normal way I used to. I got to my desk and there sat an artificial rose. I knew Donna was thinking about me. I choked my tears back and tried to pretend nothing happened. I looked at my messages and sat down and tried to call my insured's back pretending nothing was happening. It just kept rolling through my mind "keep your sanity, hold on Cheryl, you can do this." Donna came around the corner of my office, I thanked her for the kind thought. I could see she wanted to give me a big hug and I stopped her. "Please don't, my eyes have been dry for 12 hours now, I have to hold on." Her smile let me know how hard it was for her to restrain and she was backing me 100 %. Diane came around the corner behind her. Diane's eyes did the same. "I have to tell Ray I will be out tomorrow for another sick day." I pulled up my chin and tried not to pout, "I have to see a Neurosurgeon tomorrow morning. He will explain to us what is happening. For today I want to work, I want to keep living and I will ask that you help me." Both ladies understood. After that I went to Ray's office and tried to fill him in on the events as best I could. I was so proud of myself, I didn't cry.

That evening Bob was ready with the scan films. He said the tumor didn't look that big to him. Out of fear I took his word for it and continued on with making dinner. I was so tired and so drained it felt like if I had to move another muscle I would fall down. I just kept on pretending that this would pass with flying colors. We chatted about Bob's recovery over dinner and I was so glad he was feeling so much better. The twenty-minute ride to the clinic didn't hurt his back; he walked across the clinic with ease. As we talked my eyes kept on glancing over to the big package of films. Bob was getting tired and went downstairs to our family room to relax. I cleaned up the mess in the kitchen, filled the dishwasher and washed the pans. The large package of films kept haunting me from the corner of the kitchen. I called down to Bob and asked if he needed anything to drink. He wanted some more ice tea. I wiped the table with a cloth to be sure none of it was wet, took the tea downstairs to Bob and returned to our kitchen.

Slowly I pulled the films out of the package and looked them over. The first few showed the top of my head. It looked fine there. I was afraid of finding something there that would affect my motor skills. The next film showed a small white spot. The next showed it getting bigger, and in succession the spot became quite large. The measurements on the films were saying something in medical terms that blurred in my mind. After that I figured out what the equations were and pulled out a film that showed the exact equation. There it was, a tumor, bigger than I had imagined. It was the size of a tennis ball. Suddenly I cried out "Bob, did you look at these?" He came upstairs and said, "Yes, I don't see what the urgency is." "Take a look at this, honey." I grabbed the tape measure from our junk drawer. "It's the size of a tennis ball in there!" He looked completely shocked. "Oh boy, no wonder you have been feeling so rotten." That completely was an understatement. He had no clue what I was feeling for the past few months, I had been hiding it. My hands started to tremble. I started once again to cover it up, "No wonder my eyes hurt, my head hurts and the headaches are so bad. What is that thing lurking inside my head?" We were both speechless looking at the MRI films. I don't know what Bob was thinking, at that point I was so consumed with fear it didn't seem to matter anymore. I cared what was going to happen, I cared about him and our girls, but my thoughts turned to me and how I was to start planning to get prepared for the worst.

Bob held me close, like he could feel what I was thinking. "We are going to get through this, I am not going to lose you." I could feel and hear the fear in his voice. "We have to talk to the doctor tomorrow and take it from there. Letting our fear get in the way will not help." Oh how I wished you could take it away, the fear, the trauma of knowing these things. I can't pray the tumor away, I can't wish it away, and I can't do anything right now but hope I can live. Of all the things a person can hear that are terrible, one is a bad heart, the other is a lung and the other is brain and a tumor. Such a touchy place to operate, all of my organs can be affected, or one of my organs can be affected, or some of them. My motor skills, my speech, my sight, my senses of touch, all of those thoughts raced through my mind. I stood there just looking at the films. Disbelief, anger, sorrow, anxiety all hit me at the same time. Suddenly a gasp hit me from the emotions, "Oh" I paused, and at that moment looking in to Bob's sad eyes lasted forever, "I just don't know what to do, feel or say. Please stand by me, please hug me when I need it." That was a silly thing to say. I know he will be there for me, I know he is just as afraid. How I hated hurting him like this, guilt became an emotion that at the time was so overwhelming that really wasn't my fault.

We discussed what to ask when we went to the doctor's office the next day. It was so hard to focus. What do we ask? This is such an unknown area and so mystifying the discussion became oblivious. It felt like a bad dream. When I realized I wasn't focusing anymore I grabbed a pad and paper and started to write down things that came to our minds. It felt so unreal that suddenly I had to change the subject. I started to ramble on about our past together and how much fun I had raising the girls. When the subject turned to them I was even more upset. How do I tell them? I am their mother, a person they were counting on to be there for them for a much longer time than promised right now. What if I can't help them with their future? I made Bob promise to do his best without me. He was so startled when I blurted that out. "We are not going to let that happen!" came out in a stern voice. "You are not allowed to give up and leave this to me." I retorted, "Right now I don't feel like I have any control on this situation, please don't argue with me, I am just asking you to help." He grabbed me with his big cuddly arms and held me close again. "We are both scared, we will find a way."

The night was long and dark. My mind wandered on to my past life and what I had hoped would be my future. The minutes on the clock went on till 3 am. About then sleep finally came. My dreams were full of color and life. They had beautiful flowers and the smell was wonderful. It was detailed with sweet smells, full of lavender and rose scents as I walked along the path. The dream was so full of life as if it were telling me it was something I was forgetting to fight for. My father appeared in my dream full of smiles and his favorite encouraging statement rang through my ears, "Smile, it will hurt less." I saw his smile, his warm loving face again. He was standing in front of me. I reached out to him for a hug, under his suit coat was a hospital gown. I felt his hand was warm and felt his heart beating. As I held him closer I whispered, "Dad, I know you had to leave us, I am not supposed to feel your warmth anymore and I am not supposed to feel your heart beat anymore." His warm blue eyes met mine, deeper than when he was alive, "My heart is beating to give you strength, and my warm hand is to let you know we are here for you." The dream startled me out of a nice slumber. I lay there awake thinking about the dream over and over, relishing in the thought my dad was there for me and wishing in my waking life I could run to him and let him give me strength one more time.

Morning came up quickly after that. I heard the coffee pot timer go off and could smell it brewing from upstairs once it had gotten to half a pot. I watched Bob sleep. His brows were knitted. The sunlight was beaming across the bedroom. I could see Angel and Winston waiting to come up in the bed and join us. I kissed Bob's brow softly and then a smile came across his face. He was half awake. Both dogs jumped up in bed and wanted us to get up. Bob looked at me sleepily. "I'm still here," I whispered, "I will be by your side forever." I buried myself in his warm chest and he wrapped his arms around me. It felt so safe and so warm, the day ahead seemed ominous for a minute.

Angel and Winston wanted to get up. Reality crashed right back in. I got up and fed them and let them out. Both dogs ran back in with delight like they had found something. All the fall smells were starting to cause a bird dog to want to run through the woods. I giggled at them in the normal way and poured our coffee. We sat and watched the news for a while and took our morning showers. All topics evaded our trip to meet a new doctor. A neurosurgeon. The sound of that seemed too scary to say out loud. Silently we started down the road. Both of us started to speak at the same time. "I forgot the list we started last night." Bob smiled, "Oh, I knew you would, we will just listen to what they have to say today and go on from there" He started in with how he hated to make the drive to where we had to go. Morning rush hour traffic was never pleasant. We ended up driving in to the parking lot of Children's Hospital. The man in the booth instructed us which way to go for parking in the hospital ramp. We walked silently hand in hand into the hospital up to the surgeon's office. In the waiting room we watched others who seemed to be filled with the same fears and others quite relieved once they left the back area where doctor and the assistants saw patients. I jumped when they called my name. Bob's arm went around my shoulder to reassure me.

First one of the assistants came in the room. I was asked questions about my general health. I was tested for balance. Little devices came out of the drawer to test my reflexes. Other devices tested my hearing. I looked at Bob as he sat with wonder what they were doing. They checked my eyes; they had me follow their fingers across a path. I made it half way with that one. I lost the fingers off to the left of my head. Little measures came out, they measured the area my eyes were spread and they measured how far they stood out from the socket. All of that was done in silence. Finally one of the aides took my blood pressure. I was stunned how high it was. She asked if it was always like that, "Oh no, I am just completely frightened right now." The student was attentive and was doing her job. She kept on writing notes; I decided it was time to break the silence. "So, can I go home now?" Bob smiled at me, knowing I was trying to escape. "Don't you want to talk to your doctor?" I smiled and said, "If I have to."

Dr. Meyer was not what I was expecting to see. He was very kind and understanding. He explained what was happening. Then he brought out the scans from the MRI tests. He put them up on the screen that showed what he was about to point out. The mass of tumor was the size of a tennis ball. He outlined it. Then he showed us where my skull was four times thicker than the other side. The out of body feeling was overwhelming. He showed us where the tumor was rubbing and invading the eye area including the nerves. Dr. Meyer started to explain how he would need two other doctors to help with the surgery and how I would need to see an Ophthalmologist. He explained how this doctor was so good at what he does that others come from countries around the world to learn from him. We needed to know after his visit if my eye could be saved. "Hold it," I quivered, " you are telling me I can lose my eye?" The doctor put his hand on mine, "yes honey, we are, we need to determine how much damage the tumor has done to your nerves in the optic area." I started to cry, I needed to sit down. My eye, my left eye, is all I could hear in my head. After that Dr. Meyer explained the procedure I was to endure. I didn't hear anything more. It all went in to a haze I couldn't break from.

Bob and I walked out to the reception area in disbelief. We scheduled an appointment with the ophthalmologist and then another with Dr. Meyer. He would plan out the doctors for surgery. He would go over what is happening again. We would get instructions what to do next. Dr. Meyer needed to get the final results from this new doctor. I needed more tests. He sent us to the Lab for blood tests to make sure my body could handle the journey it was about to take. I sat there and held on to Bob and waited for my turn. A woman in front of us told us her story, how she had a heart attack and how her surgery went so well. Then she began to tell us about how her now ex-husband couldn't handle the stress from her health problems and served her divorce papers while she lay in a hospital bed recovering. I looked at her with disbelief. Her mother was with her giving her comfort. They left and I was so stunned. I looked up at my own husband and he could read my mind. "I wouldn't dream of doing that to you. I am here, I still love you." The lady finally called me in to the lab. She drew my blood, six vials full. I looked down at the fifth vial, without a word. "Your doctor wants to know everything he can right now." I chuckled, "And how, gee, leave some in there!" She smiled. When she put the bandage on my arm and let me walk out I suddenly felt dizzy. It wasn't from the blood draw; it was from all of the information that went through my mind. I walked out to Bob and sat down next to him. "Are you ok?" "Oh, I don't think so, not this time," I responded. "What did they do in there?" he asked. My response was shaky, "They only drew blood and that wasn't what happed, I sat there silently trying to absorb what I just learned." The lightning bolt hit again, across the front my head that I had to concentrate as to where I was. The lights had gotten very bright and then dim and I could not see out of my eye at all. Bob came up on the left side of me. I could feel him there but not see him. I turned my head to look at him. He went blurry. As I concentrated on his face I couldn't see where his nose was to jut out and his eyes to sink in. All of the three dimensional vision was completely gone. It happened so fast, as if each lightning bolt headache made me a little worse each time. "Can we leave now?" I asked. "I want to go home." The ride was quiet, both of us in deep thought.

We walked into the kitchen and let the dogs out of the upstairs where we gated them when we left home. I loved the wagging tails and the greetings from them. Both Bob and I remained silent, just looking at each other without saying a word. After greeting the puppies I sat down at the kitchen table with Bob who remained silent. "Honey, I am so sorry, this is too much information and too much to handle at one given moment." He smiled back at me with his earnest eyes. "I know the feeling." "I have to try gather strength from here, I have to find the courage to tell our girls, I don't know how to do this." I just rambled on, "How do I tell our children? How do I tell my mother when she calls on Sunday? Worse yet, how do I survive this one?" Bob grabbed my hand on the table, "We are going to get through this, and we are going to take one day at a time while you gain strength to do this." I knew I had hurt him deeply, how does a man look at his wife with such terror in her, how does he stay calm to help her, and most of all how did he hide his fear? It was there, but in mine I couldn't feel it, the numbness overcame my emotions.

Bob went on with trying to have some normalcy in our lives. He fed the dogs and let them play in the back yard. I watched them intently. My head suddenly hurt again, my left eye completely blurred and I closed it so I could see what was happening around me. I looked at the wainscot made around the kitchen table; it was only there. I could see the panels Bob put together from the doors and thought how nice it looked and wished I could see the three dimensional effect from the panels. I pondered on it wasn't so unusual that I kept on tripping on steps and how it was a miracle I didn't get hurt. I knew this was happening at my bother-in-law's birthday party in August when I tripped on the step there. I knew the secret would come out.

When Bob came in the door with the dogs I had been contemplating on how we would inform the girls. "We should have the girls for dinner tomorrow, they need to know before anyone else. I want to make sure the boys join them to get them home safely. They will be too upset to drive home on their own." Bob looked at me with eyes understanding what I was trying to do. "How do you plan on doing this?" "I want to tell them we are having a celebration to honor your recovery. We can break it to them later, together. I will cook like never before and make the evening seem as though nothing is wrong until everyone is settled in the comfort of the evening. Make them relax, until I have to let them know I am so sick."

Bob responded and smiled at me with such earnest eyes. "If that is how you would like to handle this I respect it. You can do what you need to in this situation." I snickered, "Situation, that's the best way to put it. We have no idea if this tumor is benign or malignant, we won't know until I am in surgery. If what the neurosurgeon says, we don't even know if I will get to come out of surgery, not until that day." I began to cry, Bob grabbed me and hugged me so hard I thought I would choke. I relished in the feeling of him holding me and not telling him I didn't know if those hugs would be a limited thing. It felt so good to feel safe in his arms for a few minutes. I just didn't want to let go and it was clear he didn't either. "My gosh, the feelings are so numb and scary." I looked up at my tender man with such adoration and wished I had his courage. He was so strong for me, so supportive and so sensitive that I felt breathless from all of the emotions.

We called the girls the next day. I faked it. I said let's have a dinner to celebrate how well Dad did and enjoy an evening together. Both girls thought that would be a good idea. "I don't know if Chris can come," Dana said. I sat there in silence for a second waiting for her reason. "He is so tired from working extra time." "Please have him come with you, I promise not to keep you too long," I replied. After it was decided both girls and their guys were coming for dinner. One hurdle was over. What do I want to cook; it has to be something they all enjoy. I started to think about this instead of going through my private mourning.

That night sleep was hard to come by. I tossed and turned; I cried and walked the house to try finding comfort somewhere. Bob was sleeping well and I watched him for a while. He started to dream and tossed a bit too. I put my hand on his arm and the dream seemed to pass on for him. I hated what I was doing to him, hurting him with my problem. I hated what he had to go through wished I could just help him heal from the surgery. After I could see he was sleeping well I walked down the stairs and into the recreation room on the lower level of our house. That is the only place that if I needed to pace I wouldn't wake up Bob. And I did just that, in the dark, looking at the streetlight in front of the house because it was one of the things I could see in the dark. I stared at it for a long time while my thoughts raced.

How do I tell my children such a terrible thing? I felt sorrow for them. They had to listen how another parent was ill and we don't know if there is a cure, if I will be able to watch them get married, graduate college, have children and do my best to help them. How can I be such a mean mother to have to tell them? It crossed my mind to not say anything until surgery day, and then realized that wouldn't be fair to them. It had to be done. I could see in my mind the sorrow on their faces. It was like telling my husband all over again, this time I would have them together and get it over with. I thought of how I encouraged my mother to go to England and how she was to call on Sunday. How does a daughter tell her mother? Then it occurred to me I had to tell the rest of my family also. After the girls know.

I stood there a while longer and tried to see the streetlight with my left eye. It was there and then again not, it faded in and out. I blinked it back into sight and then it would fade to all black out of that eye. I would try to see the halo around the light; it just disappeared. The pole was somewhere connected to it; memory let me see it. I felt so fearful, would they be able to save my eye? Will they be able to get the tumor out? Will they be able to save me? Will I go completely blind? Are there any handicaps I will have to face? I never learned braille, I never ever thought of dying so young. The chills overcame me again, shaking from head to toe. I began to feel exhausted, went to the kitchen and made myself a warm milk to try sleep. After drinking the milk, I went back to bed. Bob was sleeping and I drifted off sometime after midnight.

The next morning I woke up late, or 8 a.m. is late for me. Bob was already up having his morning coffee and watching the news. When I went downstairs the dogs greeted me with their usual happy stubby tails. Angel sang for her puppy cookie, Winston waited for his. Bob poured me a cup of coffee and put it on the table. I could see his eyes filled with concern and sorrow. "What's the plan today?" he asked. "Well, we need to go grocery shopping if you feel up to it, get some festive foods that everyone likes." "That sounds like a good idea, keep yourself busy," he said. We planned what we needed to buy and got dressed and ready to go out. I changed the bandage on Bob's back and it looked good. "Think your sweat pants and a loose shirt to air that a while when we get home would be a good idea," I said. Bob agreed. We headed out the door to the store after that.

As we walked the aisles, I pondered at how hard it would be if I went blind from this. I would have to coach Bob for something to keep myself occupied. What if I get seizures from this suddenly came to mind. I could never drive until they were sure it wouldn't happen again. I would be a major risk on the road! What if they couldn't get the tumor, what if it's malignant? This could be one of my last days shopping with Bob, enjoying his company. I snapped back to the task at hand. Finding things in the store that would please everyone for the meal this evening.

After unpacking groceries and getting things prepared Bob sat for a while. He wasn't tired from the walk around the store; I think he just needed to be by himself for a while. Gather all of his thoughts and try to regain strength for me. He strolled into the kitchen and started to help with dishes I was creating. "Are you sure you're not overdoing yourself?" he asked. "No, I want to keep busy, I need to keep busy right now." He nodded and smiled and just as I tried to smile back a lightning bolt hit so hard I dropped the bowl on the floor and held on to the counter. My kitchen began to spin and I saw stars and felt faint. "All right then, I retorted, good thing that bowl is made of metal and I had a counter to hold on to!" I tried to make light of the situation and Bob wouldn't have it. He grabbed my hand and led me to the front room couch and made me sit for a minute. When he came back from the kitchen he sat next to me. "Think you're done out there now?" I nodded my head and looked at the floor. "Sorry, I didn't mean to scare you, never had one like that before." "Do you think you're trying too hard, honey?" he asked. "Are you tired? The girls and boys won't be here for a while, will you try to rest for now." I replied, "I will if you do." He grabbed my hand and we went upstairs for a nap.

Quickly an hour passed and we just lay there on the bed in each other's arms silently for a while. "That was nice, a good rest," I said to break the silence. "Yeah, I guess it's time to get up and finish getting ready for the kids to come. They will be here in about an hour." Bob put the leaf in the table and set the dishes out while I finished cooking. Soon after that Aja and Ryan came. Angel and Winston were so happy to see them. Directly after that Dana and Chris came and more happy doggy greetings came. Rico squawked from the basement until Aja ran down to get him. The girls were asking Bob how he was feeling and noticed he looked tired. I hid my face letting them pamper him. It was so nice to see how they were so concerned and caring towards their father. Both girls adored him, just as it should be.

Dinner was fun, we laughed and talked all the way through it. The girls and I talked about how Bob was so funny at the hospital and when he came home. How he talked about watching TV and there wasn't a TV in our room. He was laughing at himself for being so funny and made us promise to never bring a dancing chicken in a hospital room to him again. We were all scolded for putting the stuffed chicken that played the chicken dance in front of him in his room. We deserved it. We laughed about things in the past that were funny and the guys hearing some of the stories for the first time really had fun hearing them too. When dessert was over, Bob and I cleaned the kitchen and the kids went to the front room to catch up on each other's lives. We smiled at each other as we could hear some of the things they were saying and were happy they were talking so nicely since they hadn't for a while.

When the dishes were finally done Bob and I entered the front room to chat with the children. Or that was the format. Bob sat in the armchair and I sat on my old wicker chair across from them. "Mom and I have to talk to you, we need to tell you about something important." Aja retorted, "You are not going to tell us you are getting a divorce, so many parents do that when the kids leave home, don't let it be that!" I smiled at Bob and looked back at them, "You may wish that after I tell you this. Chris, would you please hold Dana's hand and Ryan you hold on to Aja. They are going to need you both and I am counting on you." The boys obliged. "What I am about to tell you is not easy for me and it won't be easy for any of us. I have a long way to go from here and I hope you can help me." I continued on. "I have been seeing several doctors and have had several different tests, they found out what is wrong with me and I saw a specialist yesterday. He is a neurosurgeon." My eyes started to tear up, "Girls there is no easy way to tell you this, and I wish I didn't have to, I have a brain tumor."

They both let go of their boyfriends' hands and ran over to me and held me tight. "Mom!" both said at once, both tried to start talking at the same time. "What can we do?" I looked at them both and started to cry some more, their eyes said it all. I hurt them deeply and it hurt me having to tell them. "You need to be strong now, so do I. We need to hold on and hope. I have more hope than ever watching you and your father, I want to fight this, and I want to see your graduations from college, your weddings and your children. I want to see your first grays come in and laugh at you too!" They both held on to me and sobbed for a minute and then the questions started pouring out. To the best of my knowledge I answered them and Bob tried to help. Suddenly Dana blurted out, "You're the one to get the best actress award around here, you knew all of this and didn't say a word!" We giggled around the tears. "I am so sorry, I wanted your father to get better first." I tried to explain to the girls the doctors would need to coordinate their schedules for my surgery. I will need the Neurosurgeon, a plastic surgeon and the ophthalmologist. One will take the tumor out, one will take care of the vision and the last will be in charge of making me look like me. I chided and said maybe he could go one better on me. We sat for the rest of the evening and discussed the tumor and the surgery. The boys asked questions too and tried to understand what was happening.

About midnight we decided it was time to talk again tomorrow and the children left. It hurt to watch the beautiful blue eyes looking so sad, those very eyes I worked all of my life to make happy when they felt sad.

We watched the girls and guys' cars leave the driveway together. I stood there a minute and Bob put his hand on my shoulder. He softly said, "We can't change this, you did a nice job telling the girls." "I don't think so, it broke their hearts and I am to blame." Bob held me tight and promised to help us get through this, he was shaking a little. That hurt even more, I hurt my husband, my children and they are all afraid for me.

Bob and I then went into the kitchen and finished cleaning up. The dishwasher was done and put away the dishes together silently. Both dogs were upstairs waiting for us to go to bed, snoring out of their Springer noses. Bob grabbed a drink for each of us and motioned for me to go out to the front room. We sat there silently for a minute. The dogs came downstairs to check up on us. Angel crawled up into my lap and snuggled, as she loves to. I broke the silence. "This is just the beginning, my mother will be calling tomorrow. That is the first person in the family to know and then you will need to call your mom, and we will have to tell all of them. What a rotten phone call to make! Hi, how are you, I have a brain tumor. Such a lousy way to have a conversation," I said. Bob smirked, "Well honey, you still have the knack to let people know and you will do well with this one too. Let's try to get some rest and face tomorrow when it comes." Finally I was feeling tired and ready for bed. I checked Bob's scar and it looked really well, covered it again with a bandage and we soon fell asleep for the night. A huge responsibility of telling the girls was relieved this evening and now will come rehearsing how we will tell each member of the families. This nightmare is far from over. Informing the families is only one very small part of the battle we are going to endure and as with all battles, no one can predict how long it will take or if we can win.

3.
Telling the Families

Sunday morning came in with beautiful sunshine and another warm October day. We got up to feed the dogs and enjoyed our usual pot of coffee and read the Sunday paper. It felt nice to not discuss the events that happened the past few days. The weather report showed it would still be balmy for this time of year. I saved the coupons as usual to clip out later. The TV section was also kept aside to watch out for what would be good to watch for the remainder of the week.

Shortly after that I went to the recreation room to get Rico and take him to the shower with me. He loves his showers. He expands his wings and lets the water flow over him. All the while he cackles and makes kissing noises letting me know he loves it so much. When I would towel dry he would flap his wings and wait to get back on to my shoulder to play with a q-tip. He loved it until I brushed my hair, the hairbrush seemed to be his enemy and he would peck at it. Rico was the noisiest bird ever to reside with us, until he was in the shower. Aja had us take care of him until she had a place that would allow a noisy bird. Sun Conures are the noisiest of all parrots. Such a screech he can put out! After that he went to his cage and played on his jungle gym.

As always, I finished dressing and went to make brunch. That has been a ritual here for quite some time. It's the only day of the week that I even consider making breakfast. Usually on Sundays we have an early dinner and relax for the day. Bob likes to watch the races or football and I find something to do, even sneak in a nap. It's the only day of the week that there is time for a nap. Working all week doesn't make it possible to nap nor does Saturday with all the house cleaning that has to be done. That chore hasn't been taken care of very well these days either, too tired and too much to do and think about.

After brunch the phone rang while dishes were getting done. My mother was on the line from England at a phone booth. Her connection was terrible and she wanted to call later in the day. That helped the situation for a while. The girls each called to see how I was and were surprised to hear I was keeping the Sunday ritual going. They had more questions about what was happening and I did my best to give them the answers. They both wanted to come over and I said to not come today. I would love to see them, but I am exhausted and would love to hear from them after they have finished work to know how the day went for them. Both had to study for some exams and were a little relieved they had the time. Both were also very tired from the evening before and hadn't slept well that night. I explained that Nana was going to call back, her connection from England wasn't good and that I had to let the rest of the family know. We had to make the calls meaning visit time was short. I think they were relieved to have to think of something else for a while.

Later my mother finally got through. She asked what the doctors had found and what was to happen. I said, "There is no easy way to tell you, Mom, I have a sizable brain tumor." The silence fell; I could feel her regaining her composure. "I am coming home to be with you." "Mom, don't cut the trip short, you are with your family. They aren't going to do anything for a couple of weeks, the doctors have to get the schedules together for the surgery and really there isn't much that can be done now." Mom retorted, "I am going to come be with you, you're my daughter and don't argue." That was enough of an argument for me! "What do you need, shall we pick you up from the airport?" Mom replied in a slow manner, "You rest, you need it for the surgery coming. I will see you when I get there." It seemed so bad to tell her, it made her panic and guilt overcame me again. I prayed for god to bring her home safely. I felt so awful about what must be going through her mind. Knowing her youngest child is now terribly ill. Did my mother feel like she was coming to spend what time she had left with me or did she feel enough faith to believe that I could be spared death at this point in my life? How was she going to get here and who was going to help her to the airport. So many unanswered questions that would be taken care of later.

Bob called his mother and told her the news later that morning. I felt awful for her too. She is over 85 now and we have been worried about her and what she has been doing. She looked good when she was at our home earlier in the month, tired more than normal was the only thing we really noticed. As Bob talked with her and the house phone rang. It was Dana calling to check in on us. I could overhear Bob as I was telling Dana the latest as to what my mother was planning and letting her know that her father was telling his mother what was happening. She was concerned about both grandmothers. Reassuring her was not the easiest thing to do at this point, but what was a mother to do? She felt much better and decided to try getting a good study time in and then getting good night's sleep. She reassured me she would call the next day to see how the two doctor appointments were for me. Bob's mother ended with take care and then hung up. She must have been left speechless (who wouldn't be); she did not talk to me. I knew the information had to sink in.

Next we decided to go down the list of the siblings, first with Bob's family. John, Bob's older brother talked to him for a while and then to me to say he was sorry. He also was left speechless. I explained to him we understood, it wasn't the normal phone call. John speechless was a treasure really; he always has a comment, joke, and a way to lighten up a conversation. He has the ability to talk to anyone, just like they had known each other for years.

Next was Judy, Bob's sister. We really felt awful telling her, especially since she had her cancer scare a couple years before. I worried how it would affect her. She patiently let Bob tell her the story and asked questions. He explained everything we knew so far. He also explained he had told his mother and asked that Judy call to check on her. When he was done Judy asked to talk to me. "I can't stand hearing my sister is sick." That statement startled me. "You never called me your sister before," "Well you have been in our family long enough and you are the closest thing I ever had to a sister." That made my eyes water, the honor to be admitted fully into the family. Judy promised to do what she could for me and asked if we needed help. I requested she tell her own children, our niece and nephew. She said I could call her anytime with my fears, she knows how it feels. I chided her and asked why she didn't depend on me at the time she needed. She said she understood what I meant. My other request was to be there for her brother.

Next came the pecking order for my family. More calls more going over the whole thing again. Somehow it seemed to help vent my feelings. At least I didn't have to call Paul; he was there every step of the way for diagnosis.

Clive, he is my oldest brother. I started the conversation with a lighthearted how are you what is new in your life? He filled me in with his life and then asked what was new in my life and asked how Bob was healing. He said he was near the hospital the day of his surgery and asked why I didn't fill him in. I apologized and said Bob wanted to just have the girls and myself there. After that I started in with telling him the whole reason why, we were pretty stressed out with Bob's surgery and with the process of what was wrong with me. I filled him in that after eye exams, doctor visits and an MRI they found that I have a brain tumor the size of a tennis ball. Another startled and speechless response, what else can a person expect in that situation? "Did I hear you correctly?" he asked. "Regretfully so, for telling you and what I have to endure in the near future." My brother, who usually has a remark or funny response, had none this time. I continued, "Mom knows and she is coming home from England to help, we expect here on Wednesday. This is a lot to absorb, and I am really getting tired. There are more phone calls to be made and I could really use a rest before I go on calling the rest of the family. Paul knows, has all the way through this mess. He caught me trying to hide a headache, and knew I went to the eye doctor to see why my left eye was protruding. I am so sorry to have to call you, but I figured it was best coming from me than Mom or anyone else. I will be calling the rest of the family later today." Clive respected my wishes to report it myself to the rest of the family and told him he can tell Toni and fill in John, his son when we know more, or even before if he felt the need. That was his decision.

Then came my sister, Jennifer. She is also a caring person, busy with her own life and children. I started the call trying to be casual. Of course she was worried I had heard something from my mother. I did tell her I talked to her and had to tell her the conversation I had with our mother. I asked how the kids were and how Eddy was; everything was fine on her end of the world. I informed her that Mom was coming home to our house Wednesday. Then I started to tell her my story. I apologized for making such a dramatic phone call, but again wanted her to know before she had heard it from any other family members. At that time she was also informed that Paul knew the process I had been going through and she was very welcome to call him also. He was willing to help with the process for me. I wasn't sure when Mom would be home but was sure that she would give Jenny a call. Because Jen is a teacher, she cannot just leave what she is doing for her class and I don't want her to yet. Again, I asked that she let her children know and if they had any questions to please call. As I received more information the family call tree would be informed.

After that I had to stop making calls and take a little time to absorb myself. The more it was talked about the more fear and worry overcame me. It would seem time to stop the calls and explanations for now. Bob and I needed to talk to each other and discuss how we intend on having the families involved. I preferred at this point to have my immediate family with us and not to have the rest of the family near until surgery time was near. When that time approached I would welcome them. When my family came to visit it is a lot of work for me, cooking, cleaning and I am not up to it at this time. Neither is Bob, he is recovering from surgery still and any more work now is too much for us to handle. Of course when the girls join us they help with the dishes and clean up but the meals and cooking are left to me. I enjoy making people welcome in our home and seeing them, it has been something that I have done for years. This time they have to count me out to take care of them.

We still have one more call to make, my brother in California. I didn't want to make that call just yet, that will wait until mom comes. Mark is not my closest sibling, not by miles alone but also by relationship. He can talk to mom first; she can fill him in that she will be staying with us and helping. It was getting late for a Sunday evening and we had to get up and go back to the hospital in the morning.

First thing in the morning was the CAT scan. The hospital is 45 minutes away and we had to check in 45 minutes prior to the appointment. We arrived there on time and sat in the waiting room until they called us to yet another waiting room. I had never had a CAT scan before and was apprehensive as to what it would entail. Finally, hospital gown and jeans I was called into the room. There was a huge machine in the room that looked like it was half a space ship; the ends were missing. The nurse guided me over to the bed and put an IV in my arm. When the technician was ready they would put a solution that would go through my system to target dye in the brain for the scan. He was very helpful explaining what they were doing and what the scan was for. He asked if I felt all right and that he would be back in a minute to inject the dye, after the first set of scans. He came back into the room and said I had stayed perfectly still and the first sets of films were good. He asked if I was to see anyone else that day and I said yes, the ophthalmologist to access my eye. He asked who I was to see. When I informed him he reassured me that the doctor I was to see was the one that saved his sight years ago. The injection was done and he informed me it was radioactive but I was no danger to my family and the wasted would leave my body naturally. I asked him if he wanted it back! He chuckled and retorted that no one had ever offered to give it back. The series took 45 minutes. I was so glad to get off of that hard steel bed. Even with the sheet and pad they cannot make that thing soft. They also prop a pillow under the knees to help alleviate the pressure on your back. The machine is so noisy you can't even take a nap.

We finally left the hospital, took a little ride around the city and decided to have some lunch. We first stopped by Dana's work and said hello to her and filled her in on the morning. It was very busy there and we hoped she could join us for lunch. Because she only gets a half hour and it is unknown when her turn was she had to decline. After that we went up the street and stopped at a restaurant we had heard had good food. It was a nice meal. We asked the waitress if we could just sit a while because there was over an hour before the next doctor appointment. Of course she agreed and asked if we needed anything else. We chided with her and said we wished she had the magic power to see the future. She laughed back and wished she could to solve our worried faces. Didn't really think we were that obvious, but then again the next doctor I was to see had the answer if I could keep my left eye.

It was amazingly busy in the office and we sat waiting for our turn. I chatted with Bob and kept on making silent prayers that this man could help me. So far I had been told I could live the rest of my life with a glass eye if I survive the surgery. Funny thing isn't it; I was so worried about keeping an eye and not focusing on the surgery coming my way.

The nurse called me back and examined my eyes. I could see really well out of the right eye and not the left. It would go black, the letters were a blur and it hurt my head. The feeling of someone touching my head came back again; it was on the crown at the top. I closed my eyes and pretended it was my father coming back from his grave to help. She said I failed the eye test in the left eye. This was something I knew before I had gotten there. Then I went to a room for a visual field test. Another one, the first really gave me a bad headache and fatigue. I explained that to her and she said it was normal for my "condition." Now I am a "condition." One of the many things I had been called today: patient, Mrs. Saler, Mom, honey, and now a "condition." The test seemed to last forever, trying so hard to see the little dots of light in the dome, blinking and it would appear, or so I thought, blinking to try to clarify the sight, blinking to try to see. I hated the dark by now; it was such a part of my life in that eye. Finally it was over and I could sit back away from the machine. My head pounded, my eye hurt. The technician guided me back to the office. Bob was sitting there waiting patiently; the test takes 45 minutes. He said he was beginning to run out of magazines to read.

Finally they called me into the office to see the doctor. He was a stern looking man, and his actions were too. The student he was teaching put drops in my eye and peered in. He was writing notes and listening to the doctor. Then doctor looked in my eye and I hadn't noticed he was also looking up at my scans. He was talking medical language to his colleague until I couldn't take it any longer. It hurt my eye to look from the bright light; it became teary from the pain of that light. Doctor gave me a tissue and smiled gently.

Come look at the scans, it shows that the tumor is now in you're optic area and we will be working very hard to not sever the nerve, I can do it so that we can save the eye. I sighed at the same time as Bob. "Please say that again, you can save my eye?" "Yes, it will be tricky but I have done this surgery a couple of times before and I believe I can." He began to show us how the tumor was wrapped into the optic area and how he will be in surgery once the neurosurgeon had gotten most of the tumor out. He will do everything he can to restore the sight but it may be difficult because the tumor was choking the optic nerves. We again looked at the films with disbelief. How did that thing get there? Why did it get so big without anyone noticing that I was having a problem? I cannot say how many doctors I have told about the headaches and the constant feelings of fatigue. The doctor reassured us that they couldn't know until something happens with the sight, or like I was getting a protruding eye. It all made sense but it didn't stop me from feeling angry for all the doctor visits made. For years I was told to calm down, don't let stress get to me, Stress! I was told I was imagining things, Stress! For hours it reeled through my mind, how could anyone think I was stressed, imagining things, not sure what I was talking about. Well guess what, this was a stress that was beyond belief, only if you have to live through this situation will you ever know true stress.

We left the office. I kept tapping Bob on the leg to the point of being annoying. "They can save my eye!" It was total disbelief. It had been an entire week of learning and accepting my life may be spent looking out of one eye, if I survive. I explained to Bob the tests and we reviewed the information gathered during the day. It was so much to absorb. Suddenly I turned to Bob at the stoplight and gave him a kiss on the cheek. "What was that for?" "Because, you are here for me and I thank you."

Tuesday I went back to work. I informed Diane how the weekend went and all about the latest tests. She was very attentive and supporting in her normal way. We discussed the whole procedure so far. Again she wanted to know what I needed. I just chuckled and said a good night's rest. That isn't going to happen for a while. Later that day Amy joined us for the afternoon break. She was too tired to walk this time, her baby was wearing on her, we didn't know what she was carrying but she sure did have a hard time with the pregnancy. Amy was doing her normal filling us in on her progress and trying to eat just crackers because that was the only thing she could handle at the time. Now, Amy is one of those very blunt people, which I appreciate, you know what she is thinking and how she is feeling, making her easy to respond to. She filled us in on how her doctor thinks she is doing fine but she has to rest. That is an easy thing to do in the first trimester of pregnancy, sleep. Then she stopped suddenly and looked at me, squarely in the eyes. "Stop hiding, tell me what is happening with you." Diane snickered, she loved the way Amy pulled her punches. I filled her in, she grabbed me and hugged so tight I thought I would choke. "Damn it, you are going to survive and be well again, and I won't have it any other way!" Amy grabbed tighter and started to cry. "Stop it, be patient with me when I whine about this and be there for me." That was the only comment I could come up with. She stepped back, looked at me and jokingly tapped my cheek. "Don't be stupid, I'm here for you all the way lady." We smiled at each other. Diane broke in, "Boy, am I glad that is over with, I hated holding that secret." Amy looked at me strangely. "Please understand, my family had to know first, then I could let you know. Now the rest of the office has to learn about this. I plan on talking to Ray after break, but first you had to know because you are a close friend in this office. I also wanted to be sure you and my new niece or nephew will be fine."

After that break we went into the office and I went to my boss' office. I gave him the story, that indeed I was sick and will be for a while. He listened to my story with complete compassion and understanding. I could take the time I needed and the company would hold my position until I had recovered. Remember that notation; hold my position until I had recovered.

The trip home seemed too long. I so wanted to be with Bob and just be home. The farms, antique store and fall colors became oblique. I just wanted to get home. I tried to make sure I didn't drive too fast; I tried so hard to pay attention to the road. I wanted to get home; to maybe a place I could feel safe. It dawned on me that wasn't a safe place anymore either; it was a familiar place to go to be with familiar things.

Once I finally walked in the door Bob was busy making dinner. He usually did when I worked and he was home first. It smelled so good and the thought of not having too much more to finish for the day was nice. We finished dinner and did the dishes together. It seemed like a good evening to sit and relax. About an hour after dinner my mother called and said she was on the way to our home. Mom didn't unpack between the trips, just took in a night's sleep to catch back up on the time change. She arrived about 7:30 p.m. That was one huge hug when she came in the door. Mom settled into the spare bedroom and sat with us for the rest of the evening. She went over the things we had found out so far and filled us in on her trip. We really didn't expect her to be at our house so soon, but the timing was good. She gave my sister a quick call to let her know she made it safely to our house. The dogs were so happy they had a buddy to sit with on the couch; they just love all the affection she will hand out to them.

The next day I had called in sick. It was a late night and a stressful day. It seemed as though I just needed a day to take some time out. Bob slept in and felt much better as his healing went along. Mom got up and started in cleaning and helping around the house. She sent me off to bed for a nap after lunch and demanded I get my rest. Moms, they seem to know what we need. Bob came upstairs and lay down for a while too.

I thanked him for letting my mother stay with us. He smirked at me, knowing we could use the help now.

The next couple of days were spent trying to catch up with all of the news from England and trying to get things ready for the family to come. This time my mother was there to help. My family gradually filtered in and out trying to say something that would ease our minds. It was horrible to watch them so upset and trying to not act that way in front of me. They joked and talked in the usual manner and then would think of a question they had about my "condition" and then would go back to the casual talk as if we could see the information had to be absorbed. Each time we talked about it they would go into thought and seem like they didn't hear what was said. Every time Bob or myself tried to get up and do a little picking up or serve someone they would jump up and get it themselves or take over the chores. At one point Bob and I were standing in the kitchen when this happened, we looked at each other with a smile on our faces telling each other maybe they really do care about us.

Finally on that Sunday evening my mother decided it was time to call my brother Mark in California. I so dreaded that call and it turned out exactly how I anticipated. My brother is in the medical field and my sister-in-law is a nurse. My brother began to tell me the process I was about to endure and filled me in on the symptoms I was having. It was astounding. The symptoms were somewhat similar to what he had spoken of but not one doctor so far told me I would be a "medical" problem for the rest of my life. It was also mentioned that it would be a miracle if they did save the eye, and that most definitely I would be blind in that eye. I informed my brother that none of the doctors had predicted this because it had to be done at the time of surgery. My sister-in-law also gave me her professional opinion and sounded very skeptical because of my age, but did fill me in on how one of her children at the youth camp had a tumor and she is doing well. At least Trudy gave a positive response and said there is hope with faith. That much I would give to her, my faith was running very high these days. Their "infinite" wisdom without consulting my doctors was something to treasure, although I really had a hard time believing anything they had to say. They also relayed their information to my mother, which I was quite dismayed about. After the sharing of conversation we had to reassure my mother that we didn't have the whole story yet from the doctors, we needed more information and neither Mark or Trudy had seen the MRI scans, nor were they neurosurgeons like that one that I had been referred to. Hopefully I don't sound angry about this anymore, I am not really, just amazed how some people can think they have all the answers without hearing all of the information nor seeing any medical records.

The following days I went back to work to think of something other than what I didn't know and what was to become of my life. It only seemed logical to keep on living my life at that time. Bob was home with my mother and he would give her tasks that would keep her mind off of the situation. It would also help him to keep busy with someone else to talk to about this whole tragedy that was happening in our lives. The first day I was back at work my mother decided to clean the refrigerator (a job I avoid) and then decided to vacuum and cleaned the main floor of our house. We live in a tri- level house, and lately it has been physically impossible for me to keep up with it. Aja had been coming once a week in between her busy college schedule and work to clean through for me, but it was impossible for her to do a deep clean because of her time schedule. It also was a good excuse for her to come visit and earn a little spending money. An apartment of her own and a full time job with her studies made it impossible for her to spend much time with us. Dana at that point in her life was not domestic, but most of all she was spending a lot of time with her new boyfriend and working over 50 hours a week, there wasn't time for her to drive an hour to help out at home. Dana would come for a visit and that was just perfect, we would get to catch up on her busy life and get to see how happy she is with her new man in her life. Little did we know at that time he would become a permanent fixture in our family.

Once again we had to go to the hospital 45 minutes away. I had to have my pre-op exam and run through a series of tests. I questioned whether or not I should give blood so that I could have my own for surgery. It was getting late and the doctor didn't think that I would lose enough blood to need that. The nurse told me that day that my blood pressure was very high. Can you think it would not be? Then she finished the work she had to do, running several tests on my reflexes, taking important information like first of kin, who do they talk to during my surgery and wanted to know if I had made my living will. LIVING WILL! I had never thought of it until now. She also advised that I decide what I should want if there would be a problem and if I should die on the operating table. Who in my family should get what, who would be responsible for the funeral, etc. Now this did really scare me, I didn't think of a funeral or deciding who should get my things if something happened. Now she was really talking blood pressure being abnormal. I could feel my heart pounding out of my chest. It hurt my head; it hurt my heart to think that these things had to be taken care of before the surgery.

We arrived home early in the afternoon and after lunch I decided it was time to get a few things done. I had to get the legal pack out for the computer and create a living will. It was a horrible thing to do and I hope that it was saved correctly somewhere so I won't have to do that again. I sat carefully and decided which daughter would get which one of my rings, which piece of jewelry and wrote it all down. I decided that if the surgery rendered me incapable and to be a permanent burden that Bob would have the right to end my life, after consultation from that doctors and discussing it with my children. I made it clear that it would be wrong for my family to suffer financially for my care and that I wanted them to go on with their lives. I even gave Bob permission to remarry because we are young enough to enjoy another's company should something tragic happen. I decided that day also to write letters to Bob, Dana, Aja and my mother.

In each of the letters I tried to explain to my husband and children that they had been the most meaningful people in my life. I asked each of them to carry on with a normal life if something terrible should happen and requested that they take care of each other. Each letter thanked them for being such wonderful people to know and each letter explained how hard I was willing to fight to come back to them. I gave all of the letters to my friend Kathy who was going to be there at the hospital with my family and requested that they not know about them until I was in surgery. That way no one would read them before hand and not argue with what I had to say. Argue? Yes, they would, they would not accept the fact there was a strong chance I would not go home or that I may not ever be able to let them know how special they are to me.

Friday the 25th of October was my meeting with the neurosurgeon. My mother joined us for the appointment. It was to inform us of what was to happen during surgery and what to expect after surgery. The doctor explained he will have to cut the skull to get to the tumor and that could affect several nerve endings that apply to my balance, thinking capabilities and handwriting. I told him I was left-handed because he was talking about right-handed people. He looked relieved. "Oh, that will make things much easier for your recovery." Then he explained the procedure of removing the tumor, when the ophthalmologist will take over and finally the plastic surgeon to implant titanium plates, implant bone material so that it will grow over the plates and reconstruct my face. He explained that I might not see anyone for a few days because of the swelling. The doctor informed my husband and mother that he would keep him posted as to the progress of the surgery throughout the day and he will know once the tumor has been removed and then they test the cells to see if it is benign (which he believed it was) or malignant. If malignant my chance for recovery would be much slower if at all. The size of the tumor could render a temporary solution for a malignant tumor that big would dramatically reduce my life span. He felt very confident it wasn't malignant due to the area that it had only worked in the menengies coating on my brain.

The doctor also explained I would be in ICU for two days after surgery while they monitor my recovery and that I may not be able to see or walk during that time. I also would need monitoring because of the delicacy of the surgery and my reflexes, heart rate and other vitals needed to be monitored for my recovery. I should expect to be hospitalized for 7 to 10 days.

We had a list of questions to ask, compiled them before the surgery. One was how many of these had he done and what was the success rate?

He confidently gave his response. I was quick to explain I did not doubt him but this was such a scary thing to go through that all bases needed to be touched. He quickly smiled and said he would ask the same questions if his life was in the hands of another. We asked how long it would take for the surgery to be performed, we learned approximately six hours. We questioned how long would it be before my family could know what the tumor is made of and he thought about three hours. He estimated about two hours would be cutting into the skull, one hour to remove and two to rebuild the skull and close (put my head back together). Once I had gotten to the ICU my family could come and see me but to be warned I will look like a truck hit me and will be severely swollen. My husband didn't care about that part, nor did my mother, all they wanted was a successful surgery, and so did I.

After the visit we headed home with most of the questions answered. The doctor couldn't answer if I would live or become disabled or epileptic or if I could have the sight back in my left eye. We had to hold on to the hope I would survive. We got home and ate an early lunch and further discussed this "situation." As I watched my mother and husband try to gain as much information from the morning appointment my head began to hurt and it felt like someone was touching the top of it again. The piercing lightning bolt headache joined in with the regular migraine-feeling headache. I tried to see them clearly but the obstacles got in the way again. Lights, darkness, blurred vision like I was swimming underwater with goggles on and could only see directly in front of me and no side vision. A streak of fear hit and I began to shake again. I couldn't sit there and listen anymore, the questions over and over again without answers and I hated being "in the dark" about what was going to happen. Quietly I got up and decided I had to do something so I started clearing up the dishes after lunch. I didn't want to say anything about how I was feeling; the fear my husband and mother felt was enough for them to deal with on their own. Both got up quickly to finish the dishes and asked me to go sit and rest. That wasn't what I needed, but they did need to do something, so I obliged.

After sitting on the couch for a while the computer kept beckoning me to find more information out on my own. Bob and my mother were busy chatting upstairs and thought I was resting. It seemed like the perfect time to do some research. I found the National Brain Tumor association on the Internet. They had so much information for me I couldn't grasp it all. I read so many interesting stories of people's surgeries and recoveries that it made a whole new inspiration come to light. Before I got caught I decided to save the site in my bookmarks so I could go back and look and read when everyone was sleeping and not noticing I was awake during the night. It seemed to be a place I could rest some of the worries and gave me answers as to what to expect. Bob came up behind me and startled me. "What are you doing?" "Researching" was my reply. He seemed a little annoyed, "don't scare yourself anymore than you already are, ok?" I tried to explain to him it was giving me additional information. Bob wasn't happy with that response so I decided to let it go and shut down the computer.

Later that day my friend Kathy called and she would be coming to dinner tomorrow and the rest of the family could listen to her story. The very same doctor removed her brain tumor five years prior to my tumor. Funny how that was, we were raised in the same small town, and I was the third person to have a brain tumor out of 2000 people that resided there.

The next day Bob and my mother busied themselves preparing for the evening dinner that the kids and Paul were coming to and did a little cleaning. Bob dusted, mom vacuumed and I nosed in the kitchen to help. It felt so strange others taking care of things for me; being a take-charge person it almost annoyed me. I promised to sit down if I felt ill if they would let me pitch in with the activities. We worked on the preparation for about three hours and then it was time for a rest. I beckoned the dogs for a nap and they happily obliged. Before I knew it Bob was in the room telling me I should get up and ready for everyone to come.

We all listened very intently as Kathy explained what she went through. She was very receptive to the questions my family asked her. I was sitting there thinking how lucky I was to have a friend for so many years be so kind in trying to help my family. Kathy did lose some of the hearing in her right ear because the tumor rested there and it could not be avoided, she showed us all her hearing aide, her scar and explained how long she was in the hospital. Because of the location of her tumor she also explained it upset her balance and sometimes she would need to grab on to something so she wouldn't fall. It has to do with the damage in the ear area. It seemed to help the family to know more about what I was about to go through. Kathy asked if it would bother them if she came to the hospital to be with them on surgery day. They all were very receptive and were glad she wanted to be there. My family has known her for over 20 years, so a familiar face was welcome at that time. That evening she gave me a couple of scarfs; two headbands were made by a mutual friend from our hometown that she had worn after her surgeries, two brain tumors this person had survived.

Kathy needed to get home, the boys were due in after their mutual outings and she wanted to be with her husband after he returned home from work. We all thanked her for the information and warned her to look out for deer on the road she was to travel home. The girls seemed relieved to know someone who survived and had many questions after Kathy left. After searching the Internet I actually had some answers for them. Bob and my mother were surprised at my information I had given out. I smirked and replied, "That is the information I was looking for, knowledge we could all use." Mom smiled back at me and nodded, she knows there would be no satisfaction on my part if I hadn't done the research.

Sunday morning Mom got up and went to church. It isn't her normal church that she enjoys on Sundays but thought the extra prayers would help. I think she was in tune to asking God and my father for help. When she returned home she said she felt much more confident about this whole dilemma and the obstacles may leave my eyesight. Not being clear on that thought I decided it was best to be left alone and not ask any questions. Mom asked if it would be all right for a couple of the brothers come from the church (Mom is Mormon) and give me a blessing before the surgery. Bob and I decided to go along with her wishes and let them come. They turned up at our house later that evening. The bishop of this ward and an assistant were ready to give me a blessing. I hadn't experienced anything like this since my baptism.

Both men talked to us for a while and Mom filled them in what was going to happen to me on the 29th of October. They talked to me a while and said they could feel the fear that was penetrating my soul. Well, most definitely! They asked Bob's permission to do the prayer. He agreed, "Anything that will help my wife is all I care about at this time."

I sat on a kitchen chair in the middle of the front room. The men placed their hands on my head and began the prayer. I don't remember what they said but do remember saying silently over and over in my head, "God, please help me." I could feel their hands tremble and wondered if my prayer was being heard and answered. I just kept my eyes closed hoping that what they were asking for was being granted. After it was over they talked to us some more and my mother felt reassured. She thanked them for coming. They wished us the best and felt things would be fine although I had a long road to travel to recovery. The Bishop and Brother thanked us again for letting them come into our home and listen to what they had to say. We watched them leave into the night and I turned around as Bob was heading down to the family room and needed to sit for a while. His back was getting a little sore and he was tired from the activities the past few days. He needed to sit and watch a little TV and think of something else for a change. My mother talked of the prayer; I informed her I didn't hear much of it because I was so busy praying myself. She seemed to feel the prayer was answered already.

The rest of the day was spent talking on the phone with family and friends wishing us well for tomorrow. They all were concerned so I decided to make a phone tree for all so that the information could be passed along. Mom made a warm cup of milk for both of us to try to help relax and sleep before the surgery tomorrow. Sleeping wasn't on the forefront of my mind, I just wanted to keep awake, keep living. The fear of not getting another tomorrow, another day knowing I was here on earth mattered most. I let mom go up to bed first. Bob and I remained behind and talked a little about the morning, what time we had to get up and leave for the hospital. Suddenly we just looked at each other silently. I gazed at him for a while and just blurted, "I love you." He replied the same back. Nothing more could be said at this point, nothing was going to change anything unless I backed out of surgery. I suggested that, and it was not an option, you see if I didn't have surgery the tumor would kill me, my chances were slim at this point. Bob was looking tired and I asked him to go get ready for bed, I would be up when he is done. I sat there silently listening to the water run down the pipes, listening to the birds make funny sleep noises and thinking of how much I wanted to return home. I heard the water shut off and the bathroom door squeak and went upstairs.

When I got to bed it felt so wonderful to be cuddled and I cherished the moment. Bob quickly fell asleep with me in his arms. I listened for a long time to his breathing and thought of how nice it will to be able to come back home and feel the same again. I listened to Angel and Winston snoring on their beds and smiled about my doggie friends and how much I wanted to just feel so peaceful and satisfied. The winds were picking up outside and I hoped it didn't mean any bad weather for the next day and my family driving. The chill of October was setting in; the leaves were turning to beautiful colors. Soon after that sleep finally came, I fought it and couldn't win, I wanted to stay awake and remember that part of my life forever.

4.
Surgery

October 29,2002 came in a lot quicker than we all wanted. It was the big day, the day when we would find out if I would live, die or become disabled. Actually that isn't the whole truth, my family would know before me.

We had to get up very early that morning. Around 4:30 a.m. I tried to pretend I didn't have to get up. Bob convinced me how important it was. Aja heard the alarm from the couch in the front room. She popped up and made the coffee for her father. I loved the smell of fresh coffee, but that is all that I could have today, the smell. My mother heard the three of us up and shortly got up also. I don't think many of us got much sleep. I sat there silently and watched Bob and Aja enjoy the coffee, I watched my mother make a cup of tea from our electric pot that Bob had to have when we returned from England. I just watched them, enjoying the sight of them, enjoying listening to the chatter. They were busy planning the day while I was contemplating what was to happen to me. We decided Aja was to shower first, then Bob then me. My mother took a bath the evening before to try to calm her nerves and I wanted to take the last shower to enjoy the heat of the water trickling over my hair for the last time for a while.

While Aja was in the shower and Bob was sipping his coffee both my mother and Bob tried to reassure me of the day to come. They both knew that was something that had to come from inside of me. Aja quickly ran downstairs to put her makeup on and Bob went to the shower. My mother grabbed my hand, "You're going to survive this and you're going to be just fine in the end." I smiled at her hazel saddened eyes, "I wish I had as much confidence as you do. I don't know if I am coming home again and when I do will I be me?" She just sat there for a minute then got up and kissed my forehead. "I heard the prayer, the blessing you were given. You are going to make it, just believe." That thought penetrated my mind like a wish that may never come true. Bob was out of the shower and it was my turn. The water felt wonderful, full of heat to try to calm my nerves. I stood there and felt it drip down over my head then down the rest of my body. I couldn't see it from the left side go down my body but watched intently over the right side. It felt so nice and I wondered if I would ever appreciate the heat of a shower again. After that it started to run cold so I quickly got out and wrapped myself up as warm as I could. Then I went to the bedroom wrapped up in my robe and sat on the bed. The suitcase was prepared for tomorrow, if it comes. I stared at it, that little carry on case with all the things I might need. The little case bought especially for the trip to Mexico to celebrate our 25th wedding anniversary. It was for our "carry on" to the plane with the things we would need right away, should they lose our luggage and what we didn't want to go into the cargo department with the rest of the cases. I dreamed with my eyes open about that trip and how much fun we had. I was wishing the overnight bag was for that wonderful trip. Bob came into the bedroom and interrupted that train of thought. He asked what I was staring at, the thoughts poured out, he promised some day we would go to Mexico again.

Knowing that I was to be in hospital gowns and such later I didn't even bother to put on any makeup or decent clothes. I dressed as comfortably as was possible. When I got downstairs it was time to prepare to leave. Bob had gotten the travel bag to put in the car to satisfy me. He knew it would stay there until they had gotten me out of

ICU. We got ready to leave and I ran upstairs. I just had to talk to my puppies before I left. I cuddled each of them and gave them a kiss. I even asked them to pray for me, I hoped they heard.

As we left the kitchen I had to turn and look at it. My pretty kitchen, bright yellow and stenciled with teapots across the top. It was so much fun to decorate and I looked at the new knobs on the cabinets I had to have before I went to the hospital. Bob so patiently put them on for me knowing that was just one more thing that had to be done before I would be satisfied. The new kitchen was now complete. It looked so pretty and I looked forward to the time I could cook in it again. I even examined if it would be the right height should I need a wheel chair. I could work, I could load the dishwasher and use the counter top and I knew I would be able to reach the sink. I didn't say a word about that thought, just silently closed the door and decided that would be handled at a later time, if needed. That same night we went to a couple of stores to find scarves and hats for me to wear when I came home. I wanted a variety so that I could play with which one would look the best, or made me feel better about being half bald.

It was still dark outside. The trip to the hospital was silent for a while. I tried to see the road signs and there wasn't a possibility that was going to happen for me. A lightning bolt headache hit me again as I was straining to see. Some of the letters showed on the neon signs, some not. I decided to for the last time hide what was happening. Aja was talking to my mother about how they wanted to pass time while the surgery was being performed, they decided the cafeteria would be great for breakfast and the new restaurant in the hospital would be good for lunch. They chatted lightheartedly with me and strayed from what was so prominent on our minds. Bob sat silently and concentrated on driving, or so he pretended to be.

The parking ramp was bare, we could see that just the doctors and staff and a few people going for surgeries were there. The ramp was so quiet and abandoned looking. Every time we had been there before it was hard to find a spot to park. The yellow lights haloed in my eyes, it reminded me of the fog lights in England that the streetlights were made of. My mother caught the smirk on my face and I told her what

I was thinking about. She grabbed my hand and smiled. Not another word was spoken about that thought but I could see in her eyes she was happy to know I was collecting all the memories I could before I was to embark on surgery.

The double doors opened up to the hospital. We all walked through the hall to the elevator and then on to the surgery area. I held Bob's hand so tight he looked at me and squeezed back tightly too. He took his other arm and stopped in front of me and gave me a warm hug from his long arms. I felt the warmth go through me like a shot of comfort that I had never felt before from him. I could see in those blue eyes of his the fear he felt for both of us. Aja sensed that feeling and stopped and held on to both of us. She had the fear of her mother and father all at once. She tried to make a quip, "I think I would rather the original thought of when I learned of this, divorce for you two, then I would know you are both fine and would heal." I grabbed her arm and held her tight, "Honey, I am going to heal. I will be back to you. I am not going to promise, I can't make promises I can't keep and you know that, but I will be back when this is all over, have faith in me, our love for each other and our family." She wiped away her tears. "Mom, please come back to us, I love you." I started to weep a little. "I love you too, I am going to try my hardest to come back, we Salers fight for what we want, don't ever forget I taught that to you." Those beautiful blue eyes of hers became a deep, deep blue, and she had a look that I missed terribly, my dad, and his eyes became a deeper blue when he was sad, or emotional. That look came through loud and clear, just like he was there again trying to tell me through Aja that I was to try the hardest I have ever tried before. I just hugged her for a minute and stepped back to look at her again. My beautiful daughter, the girl who possessed her grandfather for a minute and never knew it.

We checked in at the counter. I turned to Bob and asked if this was all necessary. Before I knew it they were whisking me off to put on the hospital gown and start preparing me for surgery. No medications were given. I was getting worried because Dana wasn't there yet and preparation for surgery had begun. I wanted to see my Dana. They took my things and put them in a bag. Bob, Aja and my mother were there by my bed/cot. It was cold and the nurse brought a warm blanket when I said I felt cold. My family was trying to reassure me, talking about what the doctors had told what the outcome might be. I was insistent as to where Dana was, had anyone heard from her? The roads had a little mist on them that was starting to freeze. I didn't want her to drive in the icy conditions.

Bob went to call Dana thinking I would be there when he returned. He gave me a little kiss on the forehead and said he would be right back. Mom and Aja assured me that it would be taken care of. I knew Bob would make sure the kids were fine. As he left I looked at his face and could see the worry sitting there. He doesn't wrinkle his brow until he has something serious on his mind. He said as he left that he would track down Dana and let me know where she was. As soon as I saw him leave and go around the corner the nurse came in and asked that my mother watch my things. Aja quickly swooped that bag into her arms and promised she would take care of my clothes. My mother touched her hand gently. Aja kissed my forehead, "I love you Mom. I will see you later, and I promise to take care of Dad." I just looked at my child and knew she meant every word she said. "Honey, I love you more than me, thank you." My confidence in that girl never wavered, not since day one when I first set eyes on her. My mother held my hand gently and smiled. Her hazel eyes turned a green I had never seen before. "Cheryl, I love you and I will see you on the other side." It was so hard not to cry, I don't even remember if I did or not that morning. "Mom, I love you too, I am giving you a big assignment right now, take care of my Bob and the girls, I don't believe in promises, none that I can't keep, this time I promise I will do my very best to see you, not on the other side where heaven is, but here on earth." The smile barely came out the sides of my mouth, but I remember telling her how much I wanted to survive. The nurse came back into the room; she started to ask my mother and daughter to leave. My mother and daughter gave me a meek looking smile and blew a kiss. They glanced back at me and walked away into the waiting area for families. I wished I could have seen Bob once more before surgery but then it would be best at this point to imagine his face.

They wheeled me off to the pre surgery room. I lay there quietly feeling very scared and hopeful. An oriental man came to the side of my bed and put some IV tubes in my arms. I asked if he could wait a minute before they sedated me so that I could know that Dana and Chris had made it to the hospital. The triage nurse said I was waiting for a call from Bob or Aja as to the whereabouts of my other daughter. I wished I could have seen that sweet face of hers before surgery but that wasn't possible anymore. All I wanted to know was if they were safe with Bob. The anesthesiologist agreed to let me wait a little while longer and informed me my doctors weren't quite ready yet.

The head of my bed was elevated and I could see and hear other patients around me. I could see two different men with markings on their legs as to where their surgeries would be. I saw a man that was going to have heart surgery and a woman who was going to have surgery for carpel tunnel syndrome. I heard some moaning and closed my eyes to sing again "Don't give up" by Peter Gabriel in my mind so I wouldn't have to listen. I heard a noise next to me and they were taking another patient to surgery. Suddenly I had to go to the restroom and asked the nurse if I could walk myself there since this would be the last time for a couple of days. She smiled and said of course. I walked past the other patients and wished I were getting my leg operated on or my arm. I was the only patient who was getting a brain tumor out. When I came out of the bathroom and to my bed the nurse came to me and reported that Aja called and said Dana and Chris parked in the ramp. I felt so much better to knowing they were safe. The anesthesiologist heard the triage nurse and began to approach me. He asked if any of the IV needles moved on my little walk and reminded me it wasn't my last walk. It was almost assuring. Then Dr. Meyer, my neurosurgeon came to my bedside. He was so reassuring and explained his plans again. As he was talking my terrifying world seemed to change and I felt very calm. He asked if there were any further questions and I teased and said, "No, that stuff you just injected into the IV made me feel 100% better, I guess it's time to wait and see you on the other side. I have faith in you, please let me see my family again." He held my hand gently. "You will."

The corridors to my surgery room seemed to go on forever, like I was traveling the distance and back in the basement of the hospital. We passed surgery room 3. "Hey," I said to the assistant, "You missed my stop!" "The doctors had to change surgery rooms for the equipment they need, I know where I am pushing you" and he chuckled. I lay there quietly and the fear became overwhelming again. At last he stopped in front of the correct room. The nurse took me in from there. I can't recall anything she said, just the green walls and gowns surrounding me. The anesthesiologist came up behind me and introduced himself. I can't even remember what he looked like. He asked if I had any questions and said he would see me in recovery. As he was putting another IV bag on the pole and put a mask on my face I asked if he could please make sure I can wake up after this. He smiled and that is the last I remember of that October morning.

My family tells me that they didn't hear anything until 1 p.m. when the surgeon went to my family and told them he had finally cut through my skull. I guess I was the first to break a blade because the skull was so thick. Three hours into my surgery someone came out and told my family that I was in recovery. That terrified them because they were warned it would take 6 hours at the very least unless there was something terrible and they couldn't go any further with the surgery and I would be gone. My daughter didn't think this sounded right and in her shock asked the family attendant who was in the surgery room or if the name was Saler. It was the wrong name, and my daughter cried with relief. Not thinking I had to endure more but knowing the doctors were still working on me. When the doctor finally came and talked to them he said that he spent all of that time cutting into the skull. It was much thicker than he anticipated.

My family had to wait another three hours before the doctor visited them again. He explained the "octopus" legs that extended around my skull popped right out and didn't give him trouble like he anticipated. He did find the "Tennis ball" in the head immediately but had to lift the legs off first. They also found that the tumor had extended itself into my cheek muscle and had to take it out from there and repair the muscles. At that time he informed my family that the ophthalmologist was working on removing the mass from around my optic area. He would report back to them as soon as they know if the tumor was benign as believed or malignant.

Another two hours went by and they let my family know the tumor was indeed benign. What a relief for them to hear. The ophthalmologist had come to tell my family that he managed to get most of the tumor out but had to leave behind a pea size amount so that it wouldn't render me blind in that eye. He reported his part of the job was time consuming because of the size of the area and amount the demon had decided to penetrate the optic area.

Another hour later my family learned that they were closing my head and putting in the titanium plates. They also had to use bone fragments from a cadaver to apply that to my plates so it would grow around them and my forehead would have its normal shape. This part of the surgery required a plastic surgeon to work with a neurosurgeon. It took another five hours to finish this project. Sewing, repairing, pasting, and putting fifty-two little titanium screws to secure four mesh titanium plates on the left side of my head. Finally the doctors came out and informed my family that I survived the surgery and they were taking me to recovery.

The first face I saw was Dr. Meyer after my surgery. He told me everything went well and that's about all I could remember what he had to say. He said my family was waiting but before I could go to ICU they needed to take another CAT scan. Because of the medications time was not an issue for me, can't place how long I was in recovery or can I remember how long it took to get to the scan area. I remember falling back to sleep relieved that I woke up to see people again. Then they had me on the gurney waiting for the machine. I could hear chatter around me but couldn't make out any conversations. I do remember one technician telling another to hurry with the person before me because of the necessity to get me into ICU. I mumbled take care of that person ahead of me and fell back to sleep. Then I was awoken with them placing pillows beside both sides of my head and under my knees. The pillows hurt my head and I moved my hands up to protect it. That was the first time I felt the bandages. They quickly grabbed my hands and apologized for hurting me. Then into the machine I went. I lay there still as could be and listened to the loud whirring sound as the scan machine took pictures. Finally they pulled me out of the machine and started on the way to ICU to monitor me. The nurses worked feverishly putting tubes back in my arms, things on my fingers to monitor my heart, lungs and any other vital organ that could be monitored. As she was working I asked if my family was near, I so wanted to see them. I wanted to smile at Bob, Dana and Aja to let them know I made it this far. She informed me they were waiting and needed to make sure everything was as the doctor ordered before they could come see me. Dr. Meyer showed up shortly after, checked on me and finally said it was fine for the family to come in three at a time. He was concerned too many would be a commotion for someone in my condition. He smiled and said I was doing well and was surprised to see me smile at him. I thanked him for working so hard. He informed the nurse he would be on call that night and to let him know of any changes in my condition.

Finally, the nurse said she called the waiting area where Bob, Dana & Aja were waiting to come see me. By this time it was already after nine p.m. My poor family had waited all day to be able to see me; anxious to see what I would look like. The doctor told us that I would look like a truck had hit me and that my eyes would be swollen shut from the massive amount of work that had done to my face. I was so excited that I could see, even though it was an ICU room. It was so thrilling to me that I would be able to see the faces that meant the most to me in the world.

The looks on those beautiful faces were priceless! When they walked in the door the bed was propped up so that I was almost in a sitting position. It was to help the swelling that would occur and ease the pressure on the head so the pain would be manageable. Those smiles mixed with tears are something a person cannot forget no matter how many painkillers were injected into me. First Bob approached the bed and kissed my forehead. Then the girls kissed my cheek from the other side. My smile was as wide as it could get, the new wounds made it a little hard. "I made it! I can see all of you smiling at me!" The tears welled up in the girls' eyes as I looked at them. "Yes mom, you came back to us. How are you feeling? Are you ok?" they asked. Bob said, "Calm down, mom may not be ready to talk much just yet." My head turned slowly towards him, "Honey, how are you?" "So much better now to see that you're here, I was so afraid for you. We thought we would see a swollen face and there it is, just a cap on your little head and your eyes aren't swollen shut." He held my hand gingerly where the IV tubes were. "Well, not to get a pity party going here, but my head hurts like the dickens!" They all chuckled at me.

Bob, Dana & Aja gave me the stories of the day on what they went through. It was so good to hear their voices. I scolded Dana about making me worry in the morning. "Mom, it worked out for the best, I was late for Dad's surgery too and look how successful it was because I wasn't here. Superstitious I know, but it worked out right and that is all that matters." That drew a smile from me and I knew she just couldn't be there in the beginning in case it was good-bye. Aja was chattering behind me with her father and I asked her to stop it. Too many noises at once were a little difficult right now for the brain to capture it all. She turned and smiled and Bob, "Mom's back." Aja informed me how they lost me at one point of the day in the hospital and really they changed surgery rooms and she chattered on in her nervous way about the whole day. Both of my girls have a very chipper voice and can chatter like, well, girls. The nurse decided that I had better get the next group of people in then get some rest. As she said that I realized that I was getting a little tired and wanted to see my mother and brother too. Bob kissed my cheek and then said sorry thinking it would hurt me. Dana and Aja did the same. "Your kisses could never hurt, can I steal a hug too? Just don't pop out the tubes!" Bob said he better run because suddenly since his nerves calmed down he had to use the restroom, I said he could use the one right behind me! He giggled at me, "You have been looking around too! I can't use that room honey, it's for you and also there is no door." Oh I giggled, feeling loopy, I can't use the room either, not until that little bag attached to me is gone!" The kids laughed, so did Bob, seems I sounded a little like I was drugged, which of course I was. They hugged me and promised to be back to see me in the morning. "Promise you will drive safely so that you can come back tomorrow and Dana tell Chris hi for me and thanks for being there with you."

Next in came my Mother, Paul and Diana. My mom gently grabbed my hand looked at my head and smiled and started to speak softly to me. "Hey Mom! I made it!" I was so excited at that time I wasn't even considering the recovery or the fact that I really did have a long way to go. "Aunty Cheryl, I was so worried about you and look at you!" Diana's eyes started to tear up. "Honey, it's ok now, don't be afraid anymore, you're going to help me get better and it means so much to me that you were here with your dad and my mom and Bob and the girls. Being here showed me just how much you care. Although it would have been more fun to talk to you today." She giggled just like the 16-year-old girl she was. Mom said, "Easy honey, don't get too excited, your machine is beeping." The nurse turned to her, "It's ok, and that's a good beep." Mom's eyes got teary too. I gazed into her hazel eyes and asked her to not worry anymore. "Mom, I love you too, thanks, now it's time for you to help me get better. I am so glad you are with Bob and helping him." Paul reached to my hand, "Little sister, I knew you could do it!" His face was so tense looking. "I have to thank you too, you knew from the beginning what was happening to me and stood right beside me. My morphine is hitting me but one last thing, you're a good brother, thanks." He smiled and started to kid me, "Nice hat!" I chuckled "like Bob would say, did they make you wear that hat?" Mom, Paul and Diana decided to get going and let me rest. Mom kissed my cheek, "I am so proud of you, I will see you in the morning." It was time for my family to get their rest and they deserved it with all of the turmoil they had gone through that day.

The nurse checked me over and over again. Wrote down things in my chart and chatted with me a little. "Your family was quite relieved to see you're sitting up and talking." I replied, "You can't believe how happy I was to see them, literally." She knew what I meant. The night went slowly. I would wake up off and on from vivid dreams. It's hard to remember the series of them now, but I do recall a few.

During one of the dreams my father came to me. He didn't look tired anymore. He seemed so happy and the warm smile he had for me went right through me, as if he were really there. He said he had gone to dance with the Angels like I told him when I last saw him. He asked if

I remembered the pictures he showed me a couple of years before. Those couldn't be forgotten, showing me pictures of the beauty of heaven. All the flowers that we loved were there. Dad and I gardened together when I was a child. In that dream he also asked if I remembered the heart beat dream. Yes, vividly. He asked if I knew how hard it was for him to visit me and be so vivid but it was the only way. I reminded him how I asked him to do so when I was at the hospital with him. It was gratifying to know he did. He cared enough to come back to visit me. I thanked him for being there, and the warmth I felt was overwhelming. He regretted he had to go and that was the last time I heard him tell me "I love you." I woke up asking him to come back. I sat there a minute with my eyes shut trying to regain the dream; it didn't work.

The nurse asked what happened when I opened my eyes. My heart rate must have gone up. I sat there for a long time until I drifted off again thinking maybe I could go back to the dream. About an hour later I woke up again from a bad dream. The doctors were telling my family they did all they could and I was floating over them begging that they could hear me because I was listening. I saw Bob cuddle with the girls and they were all sobbing. They were planning how to tell the family, I could hear them talking and tried so hard to the point it felt like I was yelling for them to hear me. It startled me to the point that I had to sit and talk to the nurse for a while. She calmed me down beautifully and I quickly dozed off again thinking I really hate the medications.

Other dreams during the night were on that order. Nightmares then there were happy dreams. A very restless night listening to the ICU people working on others, trying to sleep and listening to the machine beep behind me. That nurse never left my side, or if she did there was another nurse there to relieve her. This was the first time in my life I had ever been in a room like that where I was the patient and the feeling was horrible. I heard of a patient in a car accident, a patient with a heart attack and another that had been beaten by a mob of some sort in the heart of the city. I lay there feeling sorry for those people, wishing I could get off of the bed and go comfort them. They had me strapped right in and don't think I could have gotten my balance to walk in their direction.

Finally I could see the sun come up in the window behind me. The sunrise. It seemed like it was a lost treasure: the brightness and warmth. 24 hours ago it seemed that that feeling would never come over me again. I lay there thinking about how all the day breaks in my 45 years never seemed so important as this one. It occurred to me how that new appreciation of life was no more apparent than ever. I closed my right eye to check the sight in the left eye. It was very blurry like before. For some reason it didn't bother me, my eye was still there and I had become accustomed to concentrating on looking out the right eye. I touched my legs and arms; the feeling was there. The nurse was watching me. "What are you doing?" she asked. "Just checking out my senses, next one would be taste because so far I can tell the others are working." That nurse turned and tested me, she smiled, "So far so good!"

I closed my eyes and rested again. It must have been an hour and then I heard someone come in the room to check on me. It was my doctor when my eyes opened. "Well, don't you get an early start!" was the first thing I could think to say. He was making sure everything was on schedule for my recovery so far. As he was checking me he was filling me in on the surgery the day before and how long it took. He seemed satisfied with the progress so far. "I'll come check on you later." As soon as he left I asked the nurse for a phone. She looked very surprised. A few minutes later there it was at my side. "How do I call out?" She showed me how and I phoned home not even knowing what the time was. Poor Bob, I scared the daylights right out of him. "Morning honey!" He was obviously awakened by the phone and sounded irritated. "Do you know what time it is?" I replied "Nope! Can you please bring my bag I packed when you come? Instead of the pajamas I have in there I would really like the Scooby Doo pjs that Aja bought me. I would appreciate my slippers and a toothbrush too!" I was giving orders without meaning to. "Honey, I will bring the pajamas but I am not sure that they will let you wear them in ICU." I could hear in the background my daughter and mother asking what was wrong. "Oh no, I am sorry, I forgot how tired all of you would be, guess I was so happy to wake up today it didn't occur to me." "That's alright honey, now that I am waking up it is good to hear your voice telling me what to do," he chuckled. I could hear the giggles in the background. Bossing Bob around was never allowed and he wasn't able to do that to me either. Our mutual respect never allowed that to happen to each other. "I'll let you go, try to get some more sleep and I just missed not waking up beside you or having you next to me in the morning. I am so sorry for waking you and giving you a scare." "It's ok honey," he replied, "I think I understand how you feel."

The next few hours entailed all of the doctors that had worked on me coming in and out of my room checking on how I was doing. My reflexes were tested; my sight and they asked me questions to check my memory. I couldn't help but laugh at the memory tests. But they were very important, after all my head was open and my brain was jostled about during a 10-½ hour surgery. They needed to check how bruising was occurring in my head. I just held on to my ice pack to my head and concentrated on the questions. Later doctor Harris came in and checked the movement of my eyes and pupils. He could see the left pupil was starting to respond. He checked and checked again with his glasses that had a special magnifier on them and the bright light. It hurt the right eye but not the left yet. He made notes in my chart and said he would come see me later.

Around 10 that morning I was getting anxious to see my family. The stockings they had put on my legs to avoid blood clots were starting to irritate me. I wanted to get out of ICU and into my own room. I tried to tell the nurse that and she said I had to wait for Dr. Meyer to come back and determine if I was indeed ready. She called him and informed him how the stockings were bothering me. Such service! He advised they could come off only if I promised to move my legs about. I did that. He called her back later and checked to see if I was fidgeting about. You bet I was! My head began to hurt again and she quickly gave me another shot in my IV. That stung and it felt like fire was getting injected into my veins. The stinging sensation lasts for about 5 minutes and then it goes away. I was feeling a little sleepy and decided it was the only way to get myself well enough to get to a room.

Around 12 p.m. Dr. Meyer came back into my room. He checked

me over again. He had his little tuning instrument to check my hearing this time. It seemed fine. Then he checked the reflexes and bandages to be sure I wasn't bleeding through. Nope, all was clear. I moved my legs around for him and asked if I could go to a room. He just smiled, "We are trying to clear one for you. First they have to prep it for you. In the mean time we will get you ready for a new room and prepare the nurses for your arrival over there." I couldn't believe my ears. "I can move forward?" "Yes dear, you are ready to go on to the next stage of recovery. Didn't you like it here? I am actually surprised you don't like the attention here," Dr. Meyer replied. "The attention is great, but there are people out there who need this spot more than I do" was my reply. The nurse giggled and reminded me that there is plenty of room for others. Then it was the waiting period for the next nurse to come and remove all of the tubes from me. That seemed like forever but really it was only an hour before they were transporting me to room 516.

My husband, mother and daughter went to the ICU to find me. They were surprised to find out I had been assigned to a room. They were given directions where to find me. I waited and listened to the nurse's chatter as they were getting me ready. One nurse came to me asked if there was anymore I needed and was instructed to give me my hair that was shaved off if I chose to keep it. That baggy with my hair was the first true realization that I was bald on top. I touched the bandages on my head and couldn't believe they even kept the hair. I watched that little baggy go into the trash. The nurse asked if there was anything more I needed. I was so thirsty; the hospital was dry. I asked for some diet 7up and it was delivered to me. As I sipped and sucked on the ice cubes I was buzzing for another drink. The nurse gave me a glass of ice water this time warning that the soda may upset my tummy and it would be dangerous to put that much pressure on my head should I need to throw up. That was an acceptable thought, didn't want to cause any ruptures of the staples or damage after all that work done on me.

Bob, Aja and Mom showed up a few minutes later. I sat there and listened to them tell me how I made them scared. They thought the hospital was calling with bad news but there I was already in a room.

Most tumor patients stay in ICU for two days; my stay was 10 hours. I showed them the lovely locks of hair that were in the trash. Bob had the pajamas as requested. Aja packed some magazines in my bag, Good &Plenty candy and some chocolate. I wasn't allowed to eat the goodies for a while yet. I asked the nurse if I could have the suck on candies and those were allowed. We talked about how the day before went for them. How awful, to have to endure that. Waiting for someone they love not knowing what was happening for 4 hours and then waiting to see if the tumor was benign or malignant and after that waiting for the reports from the doctors when the surgery was over. Having to listen to those doctors and not know for such a long time what the outcome would be. We are not half way there yet. I lay there and listened and dozed at the same time just enjoying that I could hear them again. Mom puttered around me, making sure I was comfortable; Bob sat there and watched my every move. Aja just watched and then I started to cough. She ran around the bed to get a drink for me. They informed me that Dana and Chris would be in later. It was such a relief to be able to lie there and hear how it was for them; after all, I got to sleep the whole time. Everyone looked so tired. They informed me once they had gotten home it was time for the phone calls and by the time they had finally gotten to bed it was after 11 p.m. Boy was that ever rotten of me to wake them so early! I decided it was time for a little nap and asked if they needed to walk about or get some lunch. They all decided to get a bite to eat while I rested. Dana would be coming soon and they needed to let her know what room to find me in. She and Chris had no idea that I was out of ICU already. They had to know I was in room 516, Aja called her cell phone to fill Dana and Chris in as to where to find me.

I lay there thinking how nice it was to be in a "regular" hospital room. The nurses shuffled in and out of the room as I tried to nap before everyone came back from lunch. It was not a naptime for me. The nurses checked my temperature and blood pressure. Then they came in to be sure I was comfortable. After that another trailed in with another dose of painkillers. Finally it seemed quiet enough and I could at least sneak in a half hour nap before Bob, Aja and Mom came back. Just as I dozed off another person came into the room and she was fussing around my bed. She checked the trash and asked if I wanted that baggie of hair. The question seemed absurd to me but said I would really have wanted a piece of that tumor in a bottle though. It could be a little memento that I could look at and show others who would care to see what that demon looked like in my head. In a few minutes she left and I finally was able to close my eyes. When my family came back to the room they said they had only been gone for just over an hour, therefore the nap was short but just enough to try listen to them.

As I was listening to the day they endured while I was in surgery I nodded off for a minute. I heard my mother say they would take a little walk and let me rest. Bob stayed behind and just sat there silently. When I woke up the first thing I saw was his warm smile. It felt so nice to see his face looking back at me. I smiled back and he held my hand. He began telling me about the grueling day he had with me in surgery and how he paced the waiting room as well as all of the halls and outside in the courtyard just wondering how things were going for me and hoping that I would be able to smile at him again. He informed me how they lost me once and how terrified they all were thinking and knowing if the surgery could not be completed it would be good-bye forever. He was so panicked by it that Aja kept her wits and went to the nurses asking if they had the right person and indeed it wasn't me. Even though they all knew if that was the word I was out of surgery that it was too early according to what the neurosurgeon had informed us at all of the pre-surgery visits; Aja would not accept the reports and found out that indeed they had been misinformed as to where I was. Bob filled me in with all of the reports they had received; and how the doctors were good at keeping them informed after that incident. It sounded like a very long and hard day for them all. I couldn't help but apologize for putting him and the rest of my family through that. At the same time it became clearer than ever just how much love we share and I felt very grateful.

Mom and Aja came back to the room after their "walk." I knew it was a time they felt Bob and I needed to talk and be together alone. Aja and my mother started telling me their stories and I listened intently. The horror they went through. I watched my daughter's blue eyes get bluer as she talked about how they lost me and she was so determined to get the information. I listened to how my mother anguished and spent time in the chapel praying for me. The whole thing sounded so horrible for them. Again an apology slipped from my lips. It felt so bad inside of me to think that I worried them so much. After that they were explaining how they expected that I could not see them because of all of the work that was done on my head and face and there they were looking right back into my eyes. They couldn't believe how I could comprehend what they were saying and how it was possible for them to talk to me again after all of the work and time the doctors had done for me. At that point I became very thirsty and started to cough. I had never seen so much panic in my life before! Mom was grabbing my cup and straw, Aja was heading out the door for a nurse, Bob was holding on to me. More water came and after the spell I asked for something other than water. The nurse checked my chart and brought in some 7-up. The fizz quenched my thirst immediately. The pressure in my head made me sit upright and soon I felt much better. I giggled at them all, "Such a commotion over a thirsty person!" I sat there a minute and realized it was finally time to hit the rest room. My mother called in the nurse to help me, which was not necessary. I recall that the nurse stood outside and my mother decided that she had better join me to make sure I wouldn't get too weak to get back to my bed. I reluctantly let her help. When I finished I looked in the mirror for the first time and saw a very drawn and tired looking person. The girl in the mirror wasn't me anymore. She was bruised, capped with a bandage and looking rather sickly. I couldn't look anymore and wanted to go back to my bed.

Bob quickly came to the side of the bed and asked if I was ok walking. I lay there a minute and realized that it was very soon after surgery that I was actually on my own two feet. Of course everything worked out better than I had anticipated and was so happy to feel that way. My soda was gone already and Aja ran for more. The nurses were concerned that I would become nauseous and made her watch that I wasn't drinking the liquids too fast. It felt so nice and cold on my throat. It was so sore from all of the tubes that were in me helping me to breath during surgery that I didn't care about anything else until we were alerted. I was given medication to avoid any nausea, later it was explained how dangerous it would be for me to put so much pressure on my head.

Suddenly the urge came and I wanted to test my legs some more and wanted to walk. Prior experience had taught me the sooner a person walks the quicker they get better. This seemed like such a good idea. I wanted to get the blood vessels going in my legs to be sure there wouldn't be any clotting problems. I desired a nice walk. Aja returned to the nurse's station and asked if this was possible. They requested that someone be on either side of me to be sure I didn't tumble. As I got out of bed and started to move my legs felt like they couldn't hold me. I kept on hearing in my mind how important it was to walk and wanted so much to do so. My mind was telling my legs to hold me and the concentration it took was something that was never felt before, or so I don't remember. I made it out to the hall and could see at the nurse's station they were smiling. Bob was holding one arm, my mother the other, Aja went directly behind me to make sure that if I fell backwards that she could catch me. I concentrated and felt wobbly. I kept on telling myself I could do it. We made it around 150 feet away from my room and I wanted to turn back. I knew I had to make it all the way back to the bed and I did it. As I lay there a minute it seemed and felt like I had just done the impossible. The nurses came in and checked on me. Even though I felt joy and freedom to use my own legs, I suddenly became very tired and needed a rest. As I slept I dreamt of how my friend would take walks with me on our breaks at work and wondered how I did just that when my sight was so bad and I had so many symptoms. It would be an uphill climb and I fell into a deep sleep. Bob, Aja and my mother took a walk to find Dana. It was certain they were feeling happy and wanted to discuss how far I had come so far without waking me. Most people stay in ICU for two days, most can't walk for 3 days. How lucky could a person be to come this far in only 29 hours? Also, I think they needed to walk around a while too because it becomes very tiring in a warm hospital and sitting in a room waiting for the patient to come around again.

Before I knew it an hour was over and Dana and Chris were ready to see me too. "Hi Mom," Dana whispered when I woke up. Her smile was radiant, just as Bob, Aja and Mom's before I fell asleep. "Heard you took a little walk. Hope you didn't tire yourself out too much." The explanation on how nice it felt to see her again and that the walk was an "obstacle" I wanted to get past. Knowing that walking was so important after a surgery to help recovery speed up. Dana sat and told me how she felt the day before and how all of her prayers came true. She with the others paced the hospital and felt frightened all day long until they finally explained to the family the surgery was a success. Again an apology spilled from my lips, the thought of hurting my family so much was as bad as what I had to face. It was so wonderful that I could hear them and see them again. Another flurry of doctors came into my room, one by one, first the neurosurgeon, and then plastic surgeon followed by the ophthalmologist. My bandages still looking clean, my vitals were good. The neurosurgeon checked my reflexes, used his little timing instrument that makes a ting noise in my ears for me to respond if I can hear it and asked a few simple questions to make sure my brain was working correctly. I thanked him for doing such a nice job and saving my life. The plastic surgeon checked the area that he worked on. It was a little difficult for him as my face was starting to swell. The nurse later brought a bag of ice for that. It did sting quite a bit but didn't take much notice of it because I was so happy to have made it. Those stings disappear with time and that knowledge always comes later in life when you have had a surgery before and this one for some reason didn't hurt as bad as the gallbladder surgery did. The ophthalmologist checked the movement of my eyes, if I could follow his fingers and how far I could look to either side. We watched all of the doctors make notes in my chart and leave. It was time for another nap and my family needed another walk. I reminded them as they left my room to not wear themselves out because I wanted to walk with them later.

5.
The Hospital Stay

Later that day after another nap and a little snack of canned pears the time seemed to come that I wanted to try to walk again. The nurse requested that I stay for a bit and let her take my vitals, check the blood pressure again and temperature. If I had no fever, yes I could walk again. My family was looking very skeptical at me wondering if this was a wise idea. Being in an upright position on the bed helped to reduce the swelling and using the ice packs helped tremendously. Bob was obviously getting looks from my mother to question me if it was necessary to try walking again. "Of course I feel like I want to stretch my legs, it's going to help me heal!" His smile let me know he understood and how hard I was fighting to go back home and enjoy the rest of my recovery there. After the nurse had finished with me I wanted to go to the restroom and this time I made my mother stand outside the door. "I need to do this by myself, Mom, please let me try. I promise to not lock the door so that if you need to fetch me it wouldn't be a problem." As I rose out of the bed I sat there a minute to be sure there wouldn't be any dizziness or faint feelings. It was not a problem. My mother held my arm as I rose up and stood on my own two feet. "See that! They are staying right there, no wobbles!" I exclaimed. Bob and the girls giggled and Mom made sure the door didn't hit against me. My mother was so afraid I would hurt myself but that look in her eye made me try even harder. The first bathroom adventure on my own was a success. I came out and Mom quickly jumped to my side. "Do I look like my legs are going to give in?" She laughed at me. "Oh no, I just wanted to make sure you didn't get hit by the door." I smiled back at her and said there was plenty of padding around my head and maybe she needed that helmet back that she had to use when I was a toddler walking around with a fractured skull. My mothers face turned serious. "I didn't mean to hurt you Mom, I want you to know I am just fine and thank you so much for all of your help and I love you too!" That eased her and she let me hold on to my IV pole. With that I decided it was time for the walk. This time I would pay more attention to my surroundings.

We took it slowly again, my daughter holding one arm and Bob holding the other. My room number was 516, the second to last room at the end of a long hall that stretched ahead of me. It was easier this time to stand and walk. I noticed the nurse's station that had about five nurses busy with charts and getting medications ready for patients in the ward. It had a huge chart with shifts and names of who would be working them on one side and a list of doctors that would be through the hospital ward later and who was on call that evening. The nurses looked up and smiled at us on the way by. Up a little further in the ward was a man groaning from a head injury. He was shouting out obscenities showing that he was disorientated. It didn't seem proper to look into the room. The railing was nicely placed along the hall and I felt maybe it would be safe to use it this time. My mother didn't feel safe with that so I decided to wait until later when I was alone to utilize the rail. As we walked a little more we could see patients like me with their heads all bandaged like a turban and relaxing in their beds. At that time I decided to take a left turn and go up the hall without any patients. I found the rest room the family used and there was very little traffic up that way. We walked a little further and my family pointed out the elevator they used to get to the floor that I was located on. A little further up the hall was another left turn and I decided to take that route back to my room. Along that hall were rooms that contained things the nurses needed like linens and bandages and things to help clean up the room when a patient had gotten sick. There also were supplies for the janitors and cleaning maids. The antiseptic smell coming from the room was nauseating. We tried to walk a little faster past the room but my legs weren't quite ready yet. A little further up was another left corner that led back to the area my room was. In the hall across from the nurse's station was a small kitchen and refrigerator. There must have been drinks in the fridge for patients and snacks in the cupboards. I saw a few empty trays and cups strewn in there for the cafeteria people to pick up. We then proceeded back to my room and I was ready to rest on the bed again. Shortly after they came from the cafeteria with my dinner tray and smelling the food, even though it was hospital food made me hungry. I worked my way through it and enjoyed every bit. I sipped the tea after dinner and enjoyed feeling nourished again by real food. It was very difficult to eat, the work done in my cheek made it so I could only take little bites. My jaw was very sore and it just could not open wide enough for a regular size bite of food.

The smell of my dinner made the rest of the family hungry and they decided it would be a good time for them to get some supper and give me a little rest time. It seemed like a great idea, I could nap and enjoy seeing them when they returned. Bob kissed my cheek; Aja and Dana did too, they bid me a nice nap and went into the hall. My mother kissed my cheek also and I promised her that a nap would feel good. She whispered, "I am so proud of you, keep trying." Her eyes welled up with tears and she quickly left to join the rest of the family. I couldn't help but smile as Bob peeked in the doorway and blew me a kiss. Quickly I snuggled in with the pink pig Aja had given me and fell asleep. A few minutes later the nurse came in and took my vitals again and quickly left. I snoozed and tried to remember the day so far and wanted dearly to remember all that I could from this experience. As I was working on these memories I fell back into a sleep and had many vivid dreams. There were lots of colors in the dreams, some were pleasure and others were very turbulent dreams. It was as if I was sorting inner feeling in those dreams. Before I knew it the family was back and I tried to tell them about the dreams but they were busy filling me in on the cafeteria and the good food there. They were talking about how so many people were enjoying the food and how good the prices were there. Don't ask me to recite what they ate, can't even remember what I ate.

In a few minutes Aja was busy fussing around my bed, checking I had everything I needed and quickly went up the hall to call Ryan. Dana decided it was a good time to call Chris and my mother went for a walk to leave Bob and I alone for a few minutes. He was trying to fill me in on the day and I was too. We laughed and talked about how hard it was for both of us. It was starting to get past 7 and I was worried about how he was because he looked so tired not to mention he too was recovering from surgery. He reported that his back felt good and the movement was getting better for him. The tingling in his leg had left and he felt secure on that left leg again. That was a relief; it was his back surgeon that found that piece of cartilage that was rubbing on his sciatic nerve causing him discomfort. The "sleepy" feeling had left his foot altogether and it felt nice to be able to feel his toes and actually feel the sensation in the foot. This was quite a good outlook for Bob. The feeling of relief overtook me and a tear trickled down my cheek. He was a little concerned about the tear and I informed him it was fine, it was so nice to know he was doing well and such a major concern in our lives for so long. He chuckled at me and held my hand. "Silly girl, you have been through more than me the past few days, don't be upset." I wasn't upset at all and let him know that I had been so worried about him and at the same time so relieved I can see everyone again and made it through the surgery and the support I had received in the past few days along with feeling so overwhelmed the tears just had to leak out. In fact I was elated to have both of us come so far in one short month. Time, the thing we all fear, we all want more of and waste all at the same moment. I informed Bob that was what just went through my mind and he agreed. At that moment I decided to appreciate every minute that God had given to me. Not to mention the skills the doctors had used to make it so I could have more time. I felt so lucky and so did Bob. We can go on with the rest of our lives.

It was time to stop being so weepy because the rest of our children or to be children came to the hospital to see me. I was so happy to see them too. Ryan and Chris had become such important people in our lives. Chris happened along with Dana having such a hard time after breaking up with her last friend. He is so loving and supportive of her that it made me feel so happy that he entered into her life. His deep eyes and caring ways with her made me feel that there would be more to come for her. Ryan is so nice and caring for my Aja too, he is so intent on listening to every word that is spoken you can just see him absorbing. Both guys are so handsome and caring people that I could just see my girls attaching to them. Like personalities can attract to become a wonderful relationship. Personal experience has taught that to me.

They sat there by my bed and were reluctant to talk for a few minutes until I decided to talk to them. I asked if I looked scary to them, both of the boys that is. They both cracked a smile at me and said they didn't think so. I told them I would scare the hell out of someone who was looking at me. Both the girls cracked up laughing. Really it was true, a woman they saw who normally wore makeup and made sure her hair was straight now sat in front of them without makeup and a head with a cap on it and knew underneath there was no hair to cover the fresh cut up job on my head. I tried to focus on how I was able to hear them and thanked them both again for being there for my girls. Both boys showed no inclination that they felt regretful or remorse that they helped our children, mothers look for those signals. I was so happy when I saw them look at each other respectively and hold the girls hands. That gave me so much comfort that I could count on them to help my children when I couldn't just yet. I wouldn't ask Bob to do that either, he needed to feel comfort within himself to know that his wife would be fine and my desire was to return to him. Not just a body but in full spirit as I used to be. He always loved my independence and forthright statements whether they are right or wrong, it has been a standing power in our relationship, the mutual respect that we would always talk about and understand how we feel about things, circumstances and life in general. Sometimes we didn't even need to say anything, it was a mutual understanding that happens in a good marriage.

That first night was a treasure with all of us back together again. I relished on how the girls were my wonderful offspring from Bob and myself. I sat and listened to them. My daughters together with their men, it appalled me to think how rotten it was for them to have to go through this. They spilled out their feelings on the day before. I saw in their eyes and heard in their throats how hard it was on them what anguish that was for them to go through. The fears they felt before and during surgery that it was possible that I could not be able to look at them again and try to guide them in the future. It hurt so deeply inside to think I had done this to my children. I understand it was not on purpose but that motherly feeling that comes along with the territory of being a parent is overwhelming. My daughters, the people I fought to come back to and promised them at birth that I would always be there for them were now here for me. My flowers brought to me by them symbolized how much they wanted me to be the mother I used to be and wanted more than anything in the world as well as being the wife my husband needed was never more apparent than now. Those feelings were so prevalent at this time it became a main focus for the rest of the evening while I watched my family. My mind raced over memories that held us together, memories and moments that will keep us together forever.

Suddenly Bob noticed I was off in my own world and without so much as a touch let me know this. He looked at me with such caring and understanding eyes that I melted again looking at him just like I used to when we were kids falling in love. We were kids, I was only 18 years old when I realized he was the man for me and it's such a funny thing that I can look at him 25 years later and feel that way. He has shown me in so many ways that he loves me and wants to be with me. Of course we had our troubles but that is normal in marriage. We managed to stick it out and try, try again to make our marriage a success. I would only believe we have. We depend on each other, not for necessity but for all of the things that belong in a true relationship.

It was starting to get late and the kids needed to get up and ready for work the next day. I could see by the looks on their faces that they were exhausted. The day before drained them terribly and bags under their eyes showed that. It was only around eight and I was amazed how I could look at the clock with clear eyes and see that. At that point I asked my family if they were tired. Of course they tried to lie and tell me differently. First I addressed Chris because he was the mate of my oldest child, "How did Dana sleep last night?" He was honest as I expected him to be. "Not too good, she tossed and turned and talked a lot about the day and how she was so looking forward to seeing you today." I looked over at Dana, "Honey, do you now feel at peace knowing that I just need to recover from here." She smiled. "Yes, I do." "Would you please go get some rest now? I would appreciate it if you would let yourself rest and enjoy your tomorrow," I replied to her and looked at Aja at the same time. "I expect you back here tomorrow and I am looking forward to seeing you but you know how I feel, your rest and health is also important. Go home, enjoy Chris, hold him tight and know you can find me right here tomorrow." She hugged me and so did Chris. I watched them leave my room. As they walked away I scolded that they have to drive safely so that I can see them tomorrow. Both of them laughed at me and smiled.

After that I turned to Aja and Ryan. "Were you listening?" Aja was so caring also and so intent on believing I was going to be fine. "Honey," I reached for her hand, "you can see that I am going to make it. You and your sister are the people that drove me to make it to this point; you know that. Please get some rest. Go home, hug Ryan and give him a hard hug to say thank you and just let him soothe you." She understood and nodded. Like her sister and heredity the blue eyes that were so sincere looking into mine held more meaning than words. I asked both boys to make sure my girls were comforted and I could tell they wanted to do the same. It was so heartwarming to know that the girls could get that reassurance they needed from their mates.

After they left it was down to Bob and my mother. I could see in the look of Bob's eyes he was also tired. He had bleary looking eyes and he had also been through too much that past 48 hours. I reached over and held his hand. "Honey, go get some rest, you have a forty-five minute drive home and the dogs would really want to eat and go out by now." He just sat there looking at me. "It's ok, get some rest sweetie, you need to take care of yourself." I was so worried he was overdoing the recovery he had to face. He needed to rest so that he could help us all when I returned home. My mother felt at ease leaving also, and I hated the emotions I had made her go through. What a horrible thing for a mother to have to endure, a child, so ill and not knowing what was to come. My mother believes in prayer and felt that I could be saved. Bless her heart, in every sense of the way. She had given me strength before and did again. I watched those hazel and tired eyes concerned that she also had overdone her limits from the day before. I wanted Bob and Mom to get some rest and feel better when they saw me tomorrow. Neither one of them argued the point that they needed rest and were willing to let me do the same. I asked Bob to call me and let me know that they were safely home. He did just that later.

After they had left, the nurses again attended me to. All of the tests were performed on me and they came back with an approval. I requested another 7-up to drink. It went down quickly and was so soothing on my sore throat. The nurses made sure that it wasn't from talking to my family and it wasn't. They learned that I spent time listening to them. The voices they carried were music to my ears. I asked for another drink and sat back to watch some TV. I waited for Bob's call and it finally came, everyone was home safely. The phone tree gave me all of the information I needed. I tried to watch the news, did some crossword puzzles and sat back. The feeling was too overwhelming. As I lay there I tried to recollect that day and wanted to hold on to the thoughts that swelled in my memories. Suddenly a nauseous feel overcame me and I hit the button on my nurse call and wanted some crackers. She quickly put something in the IV tube and the feeling left. I tried again to close my eyes and sleep and couldn't. I paged my nurse again and wanted to try to walk again. She was busy with other patients. After a few minutes, which felt like an eternity, I decided to turn to this side of my bed and get myself upright. I sat there for a minute and learned that there was no more dizziness. I felt the cold floor at my feet and decided not to use my slippers in case I tripped on them. The floor felt so nice and refreshing. After my feet warmed up that spot I moved them to feel the coolness again.

Simple things are sometimes the best. It felt so nice and I ran out of cool spots that I raised myself to my feet. It felt so good to feel my legs holding me again. From there it seemed like a good idea to take one step at a time. The bed wasn't far away and if it was necessary I could turn around again. Another step, until I was outside my room. The hall, I made it there all by myself. I looked at my room number, 516 just in case I became disorientated. The railing on the wall was inviting and I held on to it. I walked around 150 feet and looked in on other patients along the way. I had felt freedom. It was so nice. I held that rail and just kept going up the ward. Suddenly a nurse spotted me. She turned and quickly came running to grab my arm. "Mrs. Saler, you're not supposed to do this alone yet." She grabbed my arm and wanted to guide me back to my room. "Can you please let me go a few more feet, I want to walk." She obliged and followed me. We made it up to the end of the hall. I looked at the other patients and smiled at them. I felt like I had accomplished Mt. Everest. When I turned around I was finally ready to make the other 200 feet back to my room. That nurse was so worried I could not make it. I did of course, returned to my room, and was tucked back into bed. She left and went to attend to the other patients again. I just lay there with my head above my body trying to feel like a sleep would be good. It seemed as though I reached the impossible. Prognosis was less than anticipated. ICU less than twelve hours, I was to be there 48 hours; walking in less than 48 hours after surgery, that wasn't supposed to happen for another two days. My determination to be released from the hospital became more than just an obstacle; it became a goal, one that I wished to achieve sooner than later. The desire to make it back home was a driving factor. The evening news became blurry and I fell asleep until the next nurse came in and wanted to check up on me. I gave her the courtesy she deserved and fell back to a deep slumber.

The dreams I had were very vivid again. I saw things I normally don't see while sleeping. It was eerie. The colors were so vivid and so lifelike it was startling enough to awaken me several times during the night. The dreams would be in categories from extreme fear to calmness. I dreamt they couldn't help me and that I had to say goodbye to my family to utter calm with blue skies and fresh scents of the ocean. One of the dreams I was walking with Bob along the oceanfront enjoying the smells and holding his hand. We were talking about how lucky we were to make it this far in our marriage and how much we enjoyed the years we had spent together. We were enjoying the beautiful view along the coast and looking at the little colorful fish that swam around our feet as we waded in the blue sea and suddenly I had to pull back and look him in the eyes and tell him I had to go now and how I could remain in his heart forever. That startled me so much I woke up feeling my heart beating so hard because it seemed so real. I looked around my room in the dark and could see the lights in the hall and concentrated on them so that I could see something to help me cling on to life. I wanted so badly to call him and hear his voice to know we were both alive. The switch for the light was in my hand and I looked at the time and knew I couldn't possibly call him at 3 a.m. I sat upright in my bed and watched the clock until I dozed off again.

Morning came with a flurry. Nurses were in and out of my room checking on me. One had the next dose of medication. I questioned if I had to take any more painkillers and told her the dreams it gave me were too vivid. She advised she would talk to the doctors and let them know that this was happening so they could talk to me. She refilled my ice pack and finished her duties and filled in my charts. I could hear the flurry in the hall and requested a cup of tea. The nurses were so busy that I got up and went to the break room on my own to get a bag and heated up a cup of water in the microwave. Raspberry tea looked rather inviting and there would be no need for milk. As I was wandering back to my room a nurse questioned what I was doing. I showed her my tea and let her know I felt she was busy trying to help other patients that it seemed easier to get it myself. She smiled and made sure I got back to my room and into bed safely. Shortly after that a tray with breakfast came. I was so hungry I ate it all and didn't flinch. No nausea and no problems with it going into my stomach. The nurse came back and saw that it was gone, including the little carton of milk. She let me go into the bathroom and helped an aide change my sheets and I brushed my teeth and washed up the best I could. It felt so nice to be able to do this on my own again. After they had finished with my room I went back to lie down in bed and watch the morning news. I worked on my crossword puzzle book when that got boring and felt a little sleepy so a nap seemed like a good idea. After all, I was in the hospital trying my best to get back home. It was a couple of hours later and the doctors came in one by one again. They tested my hearing again, my eye movement and looked at the staples across the left side of my face. They checked the bandages and saw there wasn't any weeping from the wound. After that they checked my chart again and notes were made, the chart and information was directly outside my door and I could see what they were doing. Every time they came to me I could see the pages growing in my chart. Shortly afterwards a nurse came back and took out the IV tube and needle from my hand. It stung a little but felt so good to have freedom from the tubes. I started to babble questions and was told that if I can walk on my own and keep the food down so well that I could go forward from here and not have to live on the IV meds to sustain me. That was another major accomplishment in such a short time.

After they left my room I decided to just relax and watched some more news. I knew my family would be there soon and wanted to get a little rest so that I could be ready for them. It was so exciting to know I could finally be off of the IV's that that was impossible. It kept reeling through my mind one step at a time. It seemed like a good time to take a little walk in hopes that it would help me get tired to take another nap before I would see everyone again. I put on my robe that was left at the end of the bed. I noticed my fresh pajamas were in the little bag and decided it would be better to change into those before I ventured on. I walked slowly over to the door and felt how nice the cold floor under me was and closed it silently so that no one would hear me so that I could change privately. I pulled the curtain around my bed and sat there feeling proud that I could actually do this again by myself. It was a little hard changing the pants, bending my head so I tried to avoid that. Success, I had clean clothes on. I immediately opened the curtains back up and opened my door again. Outside there was a nurse. She smiled at me in clean clothes and I could see she felt happy about not having to help me. As I looked back at her she grabbed my chart and noted I had done this minor feat. It was funny to me and I giggled. "Patient changes herself, no assistance needed, brushed her own teeth and washed her own face." The nurse thought it was funny too, and remarked that most brain tumor or people operated on in the brain area were not able to do this so soon. "Oh good, then I can meander over there to get another cup of tea and go back to bed," I said to her. "You meander all you want, it is getting you better faster than you realize," she replied. "Your doctors cannot believe you are doing all of this so soon after surgery. Most people are still in ICU at this point." I grinned at her, "I have never been most people before in my life and I am not going to start now. Surgery was 60 hours ago." "We don't count going into surgery, so it was 50 hours ago," she retorted. "Oh, well then, guess I am doing better than I even thought," was my response. "Cheryl, you do realize that you normally would be just coming to the ward after ICU." As she tried to remind me how serious the surgery was that I had. "Yes I do know that, and yes I am considering how I want to just get better. With a little drive and determination it will happen for me. Not to mention if God is on my side he will help me get through this." She put her hand out and extended her arm in the direction of the long hall, "Please, keep on walking and fighting for what you believe in." Before I began my own walk she hugged me gently and just stepped back.

So off I went, all on my own again. I walked slowly but steadily. I saw the man that was groaning from the head injury. I stood outside his door a minute where he couldn't see me and listened. I felt so sorry for him to be in so much pain and mused on how my own head should be hurting. After that minute I looked up to the end of that hall and decided I could make it. I slowly walked and my legs felt more and more stable as I went along. The next room had a patient and a family that looked extremely tired. The family had been in the room all night long waiting for this person to come out of a serious situation. Like sitting on a balance beam never knowing which way the loved one would go. How horrible for them. I mused about how I made my own family go through the same thing not long ago. They noticed me standing there watching and listening. "I am so sorry, please don't think I was being nosey I was just standing here thinking about how I made my husband and children go through the same thing only a day ago. I hope you all will be well soon." And I quickly walked away. It surprised me to know I could walk that fast and decided how nice that felt. It was a lot shorter up the hall than anticipated. I made it back to my room and went back to the bed and crosswords hoping I could feel sleepy enough to take a nap. That wasn't what I needed and just lay there waiting to see my family again.

My mother showed up smiling. "How are you honey?" "Hi mom! I am doing just fine, it is so nice to see your face this morning!" I knew I had a little more excitement in my voice that was supposed to be blurted out. She fussed around me and fixed my blankets and tucked me back into bed. Seeing her face again smiling meant more than I could tell her. "Are you alone this morning?" "For now, Bob was tired and needed a little more sleep and the rest of the family too, they will be here later." Mom tried to not fill me in any more; I could see she was covering something. I just let it be at that, after all I knew later in the day I would find out more. I wanted mom to just talk to me about what she had been doing and enjoyed listening to her pleasant voice. She did just that and went on about her day prior and how she was so happy that I was coherent and could converse with her. I wanted to take another walk and requested she join me. We decided to take another route and ended up in another waiting room that we didn't know was there. We went back to my room from there and she let me sit silently. Shortly after that my neurosurgeon turned up. He decided it was time to remove the bandaged on my head and let the wound feel some air. He put a thinner bandage on it and cut away at the old bandage so carefully. I could feel the air on my head. He dabbed the wound with a cool cloth and reapplied some gauze after he looked it over carefully, checked the staples and touched parts of my head for feeling. There was none, I could see his hand touch me but the feeling was not there. He seemed confident that the sensation would come back later after the swelling and healing progressed. Dr. Meyer was concerned about my walking and I reassured him that it felt good to me. With that he left and smiled in his grandfatherly way and proceeded with his morning rounds. My mother stopped him outside the door as he was filling in my chart information. When she came back I questioned her what she was asking. "Only to make sure you are not pushing your recovery." "And what did Dr. Meyer tell you?" I asked. "He told me to let you do what you feel you can and to not stop you from wanting to walk so much. I was concerned you were pushing it." I sat back in the bed again and was happy with knowing a doctor was so supportive of my trying so hard. Getting better was a goal; the obstacle was starting to leave my life.

Shortly after that an orderly came to the room and brought in some flowers from people. There was a beautiful plant from my family that was encased in a beautiful birdhouse planter. My family knows how much I enjoy the birds. It was so pretty I was ready to just pull out the plant and hold on to the planter. I still have it, sitting in my windowsill and every time I look at it I appreciate how nice it looks and how much joy it had given to me. It does sit near my live bird, a cockatiel named Norman. He was named this because Norman Bates was psychotic and so is this bird. Shortly after that more plants and flowers arrived at my room. I received a beautiful bouquet of carnations from my friend Diane and her husband Tom. There were green plants and flowers from the office. It was so nice to see that all of these people cared about me. My friends know how much I enjoy flowers and plants. Our home is filled with them. It seemed like an endless train of people filling my room. I decided it was time to move the picture Bob had composed for me. He made a frame filled with pictures of our family and another stand-alone with just him and I enjoying our time at the race. In the big picture had pictures of my family in sequence along with pictures of our two dogs. He also was sweet enough to put pictures of Rico and Norman to let me feel close to home. It was astounding to feel so loved by him and the rest of my family and friends.

Soon the phone rang and it was Diane calling from work. She was so happy to hear my voice again. Diane bubbled in her usual way and was glad to hear I could actually correspond back in the conversation. She filled me in on how Bob let her know right away that I had made it through the surgery and how everyone was praying that I would be fine. It was so nice to know this friend that had been there from the beginning was not going to leave my side just yet. She let me know she kept the whole office informed and how they were all relieved.

Next came Kathy to my room. She was in the middle of studying for her real-estate exams and took some time to check in on me. Kathy was completely surprised to see I was sitting up and talking already. She first went to find me in ICU and I wasn't there. She spent two days there. That has everything to do with the location of the tumor. I told her how I regretted I didn't understand what she went through and how sorry I didn't go to see her. Kathy remembered that was the time frame my father died and reminded me there was a lot for our family to contend with at that time. My forgiving redhead friend, a woman who went through more than she had to and was always there when I needed her and I hoped that some day I could be there for her when she needs it.

Shortly after she left because she had to study and take care of her sons the room went quiet for a while. I put my head back and decided it would be a good time for a little rest. Mom went up the hall and found herself a cup of tea and sat quietly while I rested. There was no sleep but the rest felt very nice. I suddenly noticed the time and wondered where Bob was. My mother reassured me he would be here soon and let me put my head back. She checked the bandages and looked at my staples and then decided it was time for her to put her head back in the chair and let me sit silently. After a few minutes I felt refreshed again and noticed my mom had dozed off. I watched her in the chair and thought about how hard it must have been for her. To watch a daughter go through such a horrible ordeal and wondered about the peace she might have felt knowing I was there just resting and listening to her talk and coach me through this obstacle. I watched her feel relaxed enough for a while and drifted off myself. After all, this time I was the patient who needed to heal.

Soon I heard a familiar voice in the hall. It was Bob and he was talking to the nurses trying to find out the progress I had made so far. He crept into my room noticing that mom and I were resting. I cracked open a smile and asked what kept him so long getting to me. He had been with his back doctor and told me the progress report was very good. I felt so happy for him. Of course I gave him the twenty-question quiz and felt so much better knowing he was doing so well. Mom smiled and let me know that was what she was hiding. It seemed such a happy moment it spurred me to want to walk again. I checked with Bob that he was up to it and he put his arm out and was ready for me. This time I felt so good I wanted to just keep on walking. I made him take me through every hall he paced the day before and stopped in the chapel for a quick "Thank you" to god. I sat there a second or two after and my mother grabbed my hand. I got a little teary eyed and looked back at the table and Jesus on the cross in front of us. "You know, that last time I prayed this hard it was in England asking for help with my father, now I sit here in gratitude and wish I could just hold Dad's hand and thank him for being there for me," I whispered to my mother. Her endearing eyes looked back at me. "You sat in the chapel in England?" "Every time I left you to be alone with Dad before he died, I sat and wished God would take it in his hands and asked him to not make it so we had to make that horrible decision. I sat and prayed and wished that Dad would get better, I would go back to the apartment you rented and wish I could just hold him one more time and feel his arms around me. It was harder than anything I had ever known. I prayed that you would be fine and be able to manage, I prayed you wouldn't have to hurt so bad." At that point I bowed my head, "Mom, I am so sorry to have rambled on." "Cheryl," mom said in a slow and deliberate voice, "I didn't know or realize you had been through so much. He was your father too." I held my mother's hand, smiled at her and we both understood.

On the walk I was escorted to all areas of the hospital that my family paced. It felt so good to have stable legs to take me there and so remorseful that I had made them go through all of that. It was a trek we took and both Bob and my Mother were concerned about me walking so far. I let it on to them I worked most of the night when they had left to just keep walking and trying to regain my strength. Bob smiled and smirked how he knew that was exactly what he would expect of me. My stubborn streak has hurt me in the past as well as helped me.

A little while later we arrived back at my room and I got into bed. My husband this time stepped in front of my mother and fixed my bedding for me. He gave me a gentle kiss on the cheek and sat in the armchair next to the bed. He looked tired and stared at the television. Every so often he would chuckle at the show that was on and almost drifted off to sleep. The kids came in the room and woke him up. Aja had another goody bag filled with my favorite candies. Dana had one too. The girls obviously teamed up and decided to split expenses. Shortly after that my room became occupied with people who came to wish me well. Kathy came in and gave me big hug. "You did it Cheryl!" She beamed, my friend for so many years was happy. She sat with us for a little while and said how she remembered walking the halls also; it took her a couple extra days to get going because of the location of her tumor. Sadly her tumor gave her a loss of some hearing and ringing in her ears. It also affected her balance so she will sometimes feel a little dizzy and then it disappears. Again, the tumor and where it's placed makes so much of a difference on how it affects the rest of your body.

Shortly after that my husband's boss and his wife showed up. I was a little dismayed but on the same note grateful they cared so much for my husband to come and give him support. Being in the medical field they were both surprised I was sitting up and talking to people. They brought a beautiful green plant that would go home with me. "Thank you, that was so kind of you. I'm amazed with your schedules you had time to come." Bob and Kathy chuckled at me for that remark. I let my husband explain the prior day and what he had been through. It only seemed logical, I was out and in surgery and it was not a memory for me. When he got to the part of how he and the girls came to my room and were surprised to see me smiling at them and talking we all got a little teary eyed. I turned to my girls and said I was so sorry for putting them through that. They both jumped up and grabbed a hand, "Mom, it was all worth it to see you had survived such a thing. That monster is out of your head and we can go on from here." I smiled at them both and kissed their pretty hands. Dana has the most delicate fingers filled with love and peacefulness. Aja has long and delicate fingers filled with the same passion. Both girls are very artistic with those hands. Dana can draw or paint beautiful pictures, the kind that make you dream of faraway places; Aja creates cakes in many different designs with skill that can be sold from a bakery made for special occasions.

Shortly after that some more people came in with flowers that were sent. My mom arranged them on the shelves in front of me so that I could look at them all. I kept staring at the pictures Bob had put there for me. The phone soon rang and it was my mother-in-law. She sounded happy to hear my voice again. I explained to mom Saler, if it weren't for the strong need to continue my life with her son and our girls I don't know what I would have done. That helped mom Saler to know her son was doing well. I turned the phone over to Bob so that he could talk to her. While their conversation is always short I was glad he filled her in on his progress. To me that was such a sweet conversation, to know my husband was not in pain anymore. He did still get tired easily but he was doing very well. I could see by the way he walked the pain had lessened considerably for him.

Soon after a couple of visitors left I felt a little restless. I wanted another walk and everyone was glad to oblige and go with me. It gets tiring just sitting in a hospital room for family and friends so we thought a walk was needed. We strolled those halls again. The girls asked about other patients I had seen and to the best of my knowledge I filled them in. I asked how the weather was outside and learned it was a bit chilly but my robe should protect me for a little while. The stairs were a long way down so we took an elevator ride. Through the lobby we went, I looked at the other people coming and going and watched their faces as they passed me. Some looked terrified just like we had not too long ago, some looked relieved to know their loved one was recuperating. Others looked worried and were discussing a loved one. I could hear bits and pieces of their conversations and felt so bad for them. There were also a lot of people staring at me; I gave them a meek smile and nod. Most of them smiled back others seemed embarrassed I noticed them staring at me. Finally we made it outside. The fall crisp air smelled so nice and fresh. I must have been standing there with a funny look on my face because Bob quickly asked how I was doing and the girls both grabbed each elbow as if to hold me in case I fall. "Oh my, don't worry I was just standing here appreciating the smells and looking as people were scurrying about wondering what they were preoccupied about and hoping it wasn't tragic for them." My entire family chuckled at me and said it was an absurd statement considering what I had just gone through. Dana squeezed my arm and whispered in my ear, "Always trying to think of others again mom." "Definitely!" I responded, "I can't imagine how hard it was for you three, four including mom and more when I consider the rest of my family, I was the lucky one who got to sleep through it all." A cool breeze kicked up and they were worried I would get chilled and decided it was time for me to go back inside. I inhaled deeply to smell the fresh air and agreed.

Back at my room I settled in and noticed it was almost time for supper. I was getting a little hungry and requested another soda to fill my tummy in the meantime. Shortly after that a nurse returned to check on me and gave me some more medication. She chatted with my family about how surprised she was to know I had walked so much during the day and night. Oops, my secret was out. My family glanced over at me and asked that I slow down a bit. I agreed but decided that when they are gone I will most likely take another walk to gain more strength. The dinner tray came and I shooed them off to have dinner. It was not the best of meals but just enough to satisfy me. After I had finished I dozed off waiting for my family to return.

When they came back they filled me in on what they ate for supper and I was envious. Soon after my brother Clive showed up with his girlfriend Tony and his son John. He had a bamboo plant for me and chatted about the surgery with Mom and Bob and the girls. Paul came in a little while later with Diana, his daughter and the conversation went on about how they made it through the previous day. I sat and hugged my pink pig Aja and Ryan had given to me as I listened to them. Aja noticed me reach for the ice pack to put up against my head to relieve a little pain. She ran up to the nurse's station and got a new pack filled with ice. It felt so nice on the throbbing pain. That aroused the nurse and she came in to check on me. She put another pain medicine dose in a cup and let me take it with a cool drink of fresh water after taking my temperature. There was no fever so I was doing fine. Bob was worried there was too much commotion in the room and checked with me if it bothered me. No, it was so nice to hear their voices again. The chatter was kept low so the noise didn't bother me. It was very difficult to hear more than one conversation at a time and concentrate on any of them. It became frustrating and I decided maybe I couldn't do that again for a while. Soon after the Bishop showed up with his wife. They also brought a nice little vase of flowers. It was nice to see him again after the blessing. I decided to try listening to the conversation he was having with my mother and it was too hard to hear all of what they were saying even though they were a few feet away because of the background noise of other conversations. I decided to address those who spoke to me and reply to them. It didn't bother me they were there, it bothered me that I used to be able to pick up on several conversations and continue on with the ones that interested me the most. At that point I must have been frowning, the Bishop and his wife decided they should leave. I thanked them for coming so far to see me, and how much their concern meant to me, that they would take time for a stranger and care so deeply. The bishop held my hand a said he could feel I would be fine. Coming from him it seemed possible. My mother walked out with them to chat a little more. Clive decided he had better get going also, he had to be up early in the morning and John had school. John was so quiet during the whole visit. I told him I was sorry to have frightened him with the taped head but chuckled it could be worse, he could be looking at all of the staples and half bald head. Everyone chuckled back; they didn't realize I knew that much about the condition of my head. I explained I stood in front of the mirror every time I was in the bathroom wondering what it looked like.

Shortly after that Paul and Diana decided they had better leave too. Diana had school in the morning and Paul had to work. I grabbed my niece's hand and thanked her for being here and with my family the day prior. She smiled so sweetly and repeated a statement I had made to her before surgery. "I ripped October out of my calendar, no more Octobers for me, it's a horrible month." Her sincere statement made me smile, "October isn't so bad, we have a survivor in it now." Paul leaned over and gave me a gentle kiss on my forehead. "Little sister, don't scare me like that again. I am so happy you are talking to us and walking to get yourself better." "Paul, thanks, you were a big part of this whole ordeal and gave me strength to try harder, to come back. You're the best big brother a girl could have." His eyes got a little teary and he quickly looked away. He and Diana left in a hurry after that. I could hear they met up with my mother in the hall. I looked over at the kids and was glad to see the smiling faces. Chris sat and held Dana's hand; Ryan was doing the same with Aja. "Hey Bob, look at that, come and hold my hand too!" He quickly came over to me and did just that. Both boys blushed a little. As I picked up on that I turned to them one at a time and said, "Chris, you are new to our family. First, thank you for being there for my Dana. It means more than you know that you helped her through this ordeal. It makes me so happy to see that you have made her a happy girl. I can see just how you feel about each other by just looking at you both." Chris glanced over at Dana and squeezed her hand. "Please," I continued, "don't ever forget or even think I disapprove of either of you, you're both grown people and I understand how nice it feels to be in a new love. It's refreshing." Dana got teary; she had no idea that's how I felt about her new friend, who loves to enjoy life with her.

Then I turned to Aja and Ryan. "Ryan I know how hard it was for you to come here. I am so sorry you had to go through that with your grandmother not too long ago. It's terrifying. I am also very glad you are in my daughter's life. You make her happy, and what a smile she has when she is with you. I also want both of you to be happy, keep on enjoying each other and don't let go of the love you feel." Ryan was speechless; I think he thought I was against him being so close to Aja. "Now, all of you have to get up early and go to work. Please go home because you need your rest. I love seeing you but would rather you stayed healthy so we can all enjoy our time when I get home. So scoot out of here, drive safely and let me know when you get home." They all smiled and did decide they were tired and needed some rest.

My room was now down to Bob and Mom. My mother wanted to take a little walk to let Bob and I be alone for a while so she walked with the kids to the elevator. Bob sat there and smiled. "I hope I didn't embarrass the boys." Bob retorted, "No I think you gave them a little peace of mind knowing we approve of the relationships." "Honey, are you getting tired too? I worry about you overdoing so soon after your surgery." He held my hand a minute and admitted he needed to get some rest. We chatted a bit until my mother came back to the room. I could see she was tired also and said she should take Bob home and get some rest too. Mom quickly agreed. "I think I will sleep much easier tonight knowing you're doing well." "Good, sleep tight when you get home and don't worry. I am in good hands." Mom kissed my hand and left the room. Bob kissed my forehead and decided he should get on the road with mom. "Call when you get home so I know you're safe." After they left I drifted off to sleep until the phone rang. Both the girls called and so did Bob. Everyone was safely at home, that comfort let me drift off and on during the night. The nurses came in and checked on me and I roused just enough to know they were there. All seemed to be going well and they quickly left into the night.

6.
Almost Home

The next morning there was a flurry of people going in and out of my room; all of the doctors that had worked on me during surgery, the nurses who kept a close eye on me and gave reports to the doctors, each of them checking the charts and making me go through their tests. Checking my eyes weren't crossed, checking that I had been able to hear and everything I could think of. It was getting a little tiresome and finally they came with my breakfast. It went down quickly. I got out of bed and retrieved another cup of tea from the nurse's station. Shortly after that my neurosurgeon came in with a nurse and decided to take my hat bandage off to check my wound. Carefully cut the cap around my head. He looked at the staples and examined the bruising. All seemed good for him and he put a gauze bandage on this time to let it breath. I was a little surprised the surgery area wasn't washed. Dr. Meyer informed me there was plenty of antibiotic solution on there and he just wanted the wound to breath for now. It felt so nice to have air on it. Shortly after it started to sting, so I put the ice pack back on that area of my head and face to relieve the pain. Doctor ordered another painkiller from the nurse and decided it was time to fill in his notes on the charts. He checked back in on me before he left. It was comforting to know he felt the progress was going well and I drifted off again.

Shortly after that my breakfast came and I ate sleepily. After my cup of tea I slowly drifted off again. Everyone was done checking on me and I was ready to nap again. I decided it would be a good time to rest since my family would be in later and I wanted more strength to talk to them and get back to walking. I cuddled with my stuffed pig Aja and Ryan had given to me and began to dream about when I could go home and play with my dogs again. That was another vivid dream about our home and I could almost feel myself petting each of the puppies and watching their little nub tails wag. I missed my little friends that made me smile just looking into those big brown eyes with floppy ears perked up at me when I talked to them.

When I woke up it was already after 10 in the morning. I was wondering where my family was and decided to let myself have a little quiet time. I pulled out my crossword book and finished two puzzles. Then I read the magazine that was brought to me. That got a little tiresome so then it seemed like a good time to brush my teeth again and try to get out for a little walk to pass the time. I gazed into the mirror and saw this very bruised and ugly face. My eye was beginning to swell and the bruising was starting along my cheek. The dye used to sterilize the wound area was also stained on the side of my head. I soaked a washcloth in warm water and tried to clean it off. The orange was not a pleasant color along my face. Because I was afraid of hurting myself I brushed the cloth very gently around my wound. The soap stung a bit when it rubbed against the wound and I had to quickly rinse it off. This time I used cold water to soothe it. It seemed like a dumb idea after all, the stinging wasn't pleasant. After that I went back to my bed and sat with my ice pack a few minutes to soothe the burning sensation. When the stinging subsided I went back into the bathroom to check I didn't make myself bleed. Whew, everything was fine and the bruises were still where they were before and there was no escaping them for now. The green and purple would be a part of my features for now. A bruised and battered looking woman: which I was. My robe felt so nice and warm and my slippers helped warm up my feet. It felt better to sit a bit and then off for my walk again. I went up every corridor I could find to try to pass time. I said hello to every person who acknowledged me go by. Then I began to think about how pitiful I must have looked to them. A woman dressed in a robe and slippers with a badly bruised face that you could now see the staples going down by my left ear. The swelling was beginning to annoy my staples on my temple so I decided to head back to my room and put the ice pack back on. When I returned there was someone cleaning the room and putting fresh sheets on my bed. I sat in the armchair with the ice pack as she finished cleaning and making everything smell hospital sterile again. She chatted as she worked and I still cannot remember a word she said. I felt sorry for her to have such a job and wondered what else she did in her life. Soon the nurse came back in and gave me a fresh ice pack for my swelling. "That was quite a walk you took by yourself this time, we were watching you and your stability has really enhanced in the past 12 hours." The nurse chatted on about my recovery. It was nice to hear she thought I was doing so well and I watched her put reports in my chart. I noticed how large that chart was; it made me feel very curious. What was written? Am I being told the truth?

When she left I snuck out to see where she had disappeared off to and saw the coast was clear. I opened my chart and began to read. There were so many pages of medical terms, notes and diagrams of my head. I tried to decipher a few and decided to go with her word that I am healing nicely. "Mrs. Saler, what are you doing?" came from behind me. "Oops I am caught" was all I could say. I walked back to my room and parked myself back on the bed. Morning TV was never entertaining to me so it seemed like a good time to relax again and see if a little more rest would come my way. It was getting near 11:30 a.m. and I was worried if my family was on their way or if they had something bad happen to them. They had almost an hour drive on a busy highway. It seemed best to not let myself worry so much and just wait for them to come.

Finally my family showed up! It sounded natural as to what made them late. Bob and Mom looked at each other and my mother smiled and said, "There are things to get done at the house, laundry and cleaning to do. We are trying to keep it in order for when you get home." It seemed like a good reason to be late, after all they had spent hours with me and I was sure they needed some rest and attend to things at home. Bob and Mom bubbled along talking and filling me in on the dogs and how the house seemed so empty without me there. The birds were acting up on them so they told me that Aja and Ryan were in charge to calm them and play for a while. Rico was Aja's bird staying with us and she did come over every week to see him.

Bob and Mom did not have any lunch yet so this time they took me to the restaurant with them. At first I felt a little odd going there because it was filled with people who had been to the clinics or the families of a patient. I tried to not look around too much and just held on to Bob's elbow. They ordered lunch and I had a little bite to eat too because the lunch in my room was lousy. I chuckled about hospital food and was surprised how good this little restaurant was. Out the window I could see it was a beautiful day with the sun shining on the leaves that had turned. It was late for the leaves to still be on the trees but soon the rain and winds would come and pull them down to the ground. I watched the people going past our table trying not to stare and smiled politely at me. It felt a little odd to be where the general public was again. It was a flurry of faces and conversations regarding pending surgeries for some and others about families that were getting better. I looked at them watching me and as they glanced away hoping I didn't catch them staring. Suddenly I was so happy everyone was done eating and wanted to go back to the floor in the land of the sick. Mom noticed I was feeling edgy and asked what was bothering me, thinking I wasn't feeling very well. I explained how it felt uncomfortable to have people seeing me like that and it concerned me that they had someone in their family facing the same thing. Mom quickly soothed my fears with telling me that to see someone with such bandages walking around so freely gave others hope for their loved ones. I just smiled at her with that thought, but really I was very scary looking and was so happy there wasn't any blood on the bandages.

Noticing I felt so uneasy, we decided to get back to the floor I was assigned to and let me rest. It didn't occur to me before that I had been through such an ordeal and my head showed it. The bruises and the staples by my ear had gotten swollen. The lump of staples that went up from my ear and across my head had begun to stick up like an eerie misfortunate occurrence. That it was. I had bruising coming into my eye area and the whole socket and eye began to bulge out from the intense work they had done on my head. I didn't feel a lot of literal pain but intense stinging where the surgery was done. Pain and sting are two different categories in my world. I went directly to the bathroom and looked at myself in the mirror to see if there were any more physical changes that I could feel occurring on my face and head. There it was, that stranger in the mirror. Me, no longer to be me, no longer to think so highly of myself and realize I was just a mortal person. Someone who about to be given a second chance at life a brand new outlook that I wasn't so sure I was ready to embrace.

Once I walked out of the bathroom and questions heard from my room if I was doing alright I decided it was time to look at my family squarely in the face and try to imagine what they were thinking when they looked at me, the new freaky looking lady that stood in front of them. I knew when I as peering into their eyes that they still loved me and I wondered how much this was going to change me. Life was always an adventure, a something new every day, a something I held on to and fought to keep through this ordeal. I wanted more than anything to be with my husband and children, that is what made me survive this. I thought about how I woke up from surgery elated that I could see them and the feeling lasted for hours. In ICU I couldn't sleep because I felt so happy I had made it through surgery and I was able to look at them when I was warned that it might not be possible. I stood there silently looking into their eyes and worried about what I had put them through. Hurting them unintentionally and remembering how much it hurt to tell them all how sick I was. My life was in danger: I made it this far. Suddenly a smile cracked across my sore face when I looked at them. One day they will know how I felt about trying so hard to remain here on earth as a wife and mother.

When I reached my bed Bob asked what was on my mind. "Just thinking honey. Trying to put all of this into perspective. It's a little overwhelming, it happened so fast, that tumor that hurt me for years and it had to come out so fast and here I am, thinking about how that thing almost made me leave you and the girls and how some day I will know all of what happened to you and the girls and how this will never leave us. A something that will never go away, a something that changed us forever." Bob smiled at me, held my hand and softly said, "You are here, you are what we wanted and hoped would come back to us and you did triumph, you're working your way back." I held his hand tight and looked into his sincere eyes knowing I could forever trust this man to help, be there, and we could love each other for many years ahead of us. It would be a robbery to take that away, our trust, caring and friendship for each other, a deep love that no one else could share because we held that relationship that only a select few get to share.

My mother suddenly mused about us talking. "I didn't know before the past few days just what you two share." "Like you and Dad did? Did you feel what the other was thinking and know exactly what to say? Did you both not have to finish a sentence but did anyway because it was grammatically correct?" Mom smiled. She didn't need to answer. I could see Bob was feeling restless and knew he needed to get out of that chair and walk too. His back needed it to continue healing. Even though I felt a little lightheaded I asked for another painkiller and a drink of water and decided to take yet another walk. You see, he needed to heal from his surgery and the guilt I felt for hindering that with my dilemma outweighed my mind more than my discomfort. I wanted him to be free of back pain and leg soreness, all a part of what he has gone through with discs that decided to grow funny spurs that hurt his sciatic nerve and make pain and problems for him since he was 35.

After that walk it was time for me to rest. Bob didn't feel he had walked enough yet and asked my mother to go with him. I did need to sit back a while and reflect and he knew that. They left for the long haul and walked around every place they could find. I took a short nap and felt so much better after that. It didn't take long for them to return to the room and try to make me feel comfortable. We began to chat about little things. It felt so nice to hear things that were in the past times in the conversations. I watched Bob and my mother talk and listened intently on how they had spent the time away from me and how they were tied up in traffic. I longed for another ride in my little car and hoped I wouldn't have to wait too long.

Shortly after that Dr. Meyer came back to my room. He was so kind and gentle in his ways. I would look at him and wonder how much pride he felt when he saved a life, such as mine, and how much sorrow he would feel with losing someone. He has a very calming mannerism when he speaks with you. He was never the doctor with his hand on the door waiting to get to the next patient. His astute grandfatherly look seemed to give us all comfort. His intelligence at his practice and mannerism stood out like a sore thumb. How he could take all of that medical knowledge and put into laymen's terms so that we all could understand was amazing.

First Dr. Meyer looked at Bob and then me and my mother. He started with "You did well, out of ICU in less than 24 hours and walking miles a day. Your desire to get well has been an inspiration to others who are in this ward." I grinned and it hurt my face to do so. He checked my bruising again, gave me an ice pack and grinned in his kind way while he handed it to me. "Who is going to take care of you when you get home?" he asked. My mother and Bob piped up and he grinned at me. "Obviously you have enough care and I can see I can trust these people to make sure you rest." He looked at Bob and my mother and smiled. "On that note, I am going to release you tomorrow morning. Only if you promise to rest and come see me in 9 days to get the staples out and I can check on your recovery." Mom jumped up quickly, "She's only been in here for 4 days, one of them in surgery all day. Do you think she is ready?" He nodded at her and replied, "Look at your daughter, she is walking, talking normally and eating well. I would think she is ready." Bob reached for my hand and I nodded at him. "This time I agree, it's time for me to leave this wonderful hotel and go home." Dr. Meyer smiled, "Tomorrow we will check on you before the release papers to be sure you're doing well enough, but this time I think you get an early release." With that he left the room, made notes in my chart and disappeared up the hall.

Wow, that news was unbelievable. Only four days, five days ago I was praying to survive and now I get to go back home. Bob had never let go of my hand since we were informed of how I was progressing. "You're going home, honey. It has been too quiet there and we never dreamed it would be a nice short stay here. Your gallbladder was ten days." I smiled back at him, "I warned you I was going to fight this tumor all the way, and this mission was accomplished. We have a long way to go yet, but in time we will get there." Mom gently kissed my forehead. "You have been a fighter for what you want since day one honey, I had faith in you." It felt so nice to hear that renewed faith in those two. The two weeks before my surgery we didn't know if there would be any life in me anymore and no one will ever know just how hard I fought to keep my life. I dreamt of our 30th anniversary, I dreamt of the girls graduating college and getting married some day and eventually when they were ready to let me be a grandmother to their children. For a while my life stopped, the hopes and dreams of a future because it was so important to regain my life before I could look to the future. Now, there is one there for me.

Later Aja and Ryan and Dana and Chris came to see me. The look in my children's eyes was beautiful when they heard I was getting an early release. They held on tight to me and said they were proud of how I managed to make it through this. Chris and Ryan also gave me a big hug. I was surprised to learn these two young men had actually learned to care about me already. It felt so nice seeing those smiles back on those faces. The blue and brown eyes feeling relief and willing to help me in every way they could. I could see in the girls' faces the genuine smiles return not the pleading type to hope that their mother would be able to keep on sharing their lives with them. That was a driving factor in my journey, to see happiness return to my husband's and daughters' faces. It's amazing how a young person can earn worry lines so quickly and I did see them grow on those two beautiful people and felt so guilty for creating them. After all, I am the mother who is supposed to help with bumps and bruises, whether they are big or small, it has been my duty to make them happy whenever I could. The same with Bob, I pledged to do my very best to bring happiness and fun into his life, a caring for a person that no other can do, other than his own mother. A very special place was reserved for Bob, a wife, confidant, mother of his children and his lover. I pledged to be that once in a lifetime person that would never give up on our relationship or our faith in each other. Ours was like any other marriage had promised to be, but ours only that no one else could ever touch and try to destroy. We like most people suffered other hardships but made it through them with a stronger relationship because of it.

The rest of the evening was spent with my walking and my family concerned that I was pushing myself. Never! I had a goal, to get well again, so it was the most important thing on my mind. We went down to the cafeteria for a real dinner, we walked some more so I could work off that dinner and not feel uncomfortable when I rested again. We rode the elevators that made me woozy. That didn't scare me, I want to ride again and it didn't the second time. My head and preparing in my mind for the sudden lift made it easier. After over an hour my mother and Bob became concerned about me still moving about. My energy level was high, I was feeling like a freed bird, I had actually felt relieved for the first time in days that things were going to work out. To satisfy them I decided it was time to return to my room and have a drink of soda. I crawled back into my bed and watched everyone bubble and listened as to how they couldn't believe I was actually going home in the morning.

The evening passed quickly and I could see my family was getting tired. They had been running back and forth with work and the hospital. Aja had studied in my room while she listened and added to the conversations. Dana was looking rather drawn and worn out. I could hear the chatter slow down, as if someone had let off steam and had no more left. Then I asked that the children go to their homes and get some rest. "Please go take care of yourself and enjoy the rest of the evening." Dana blurted out "Mom's back! She is worried about us again!" I held out my hand to her, she came to my bedside, when I held her soft hand I looked up at the bubbly person I know and smiled at her loving blue eyes, "Through all of this you were on my mind, how badly I hurt you with being ill, how I longed to see that sparkle in your face and smile. We are going to finish getting through this; we are going to help each other this time. Because you are a young lady now I will count on you. Remember when you counted on me for emotional support? I am going to rely on you to encourage me to finish getting better. This can be asked of you because in more ways than I can count you have done that for me in our past." I summoned Aja to my other side and grabbed her hand too. "This goes for you too young lady, I am extremely proud of both of you. Somehow you both managed to make me watch you and be so grateful that I am your mother. You both have set an example for me to live up to." They both looked at me with tears of joy, a mother doesn't tell her children how wonderful they are every day, it's something that is reserved for special times like this. And it is very true, my lovely ladies make it all worth it to be their mother and hopefully their friend. They both left shortly after that, I could see the sighs of relief and their need for rest.

It was suddenly after nine p.m. and the nurses were back in the room administering painkillers and checking on me. Somehow I never had a temperature to hold me back, must have been the need to drink plenty of fluids. My mother had taught me that. Wash your system so it will heal. It was something I encouraged our children to do also. It was very apparent that Bob and Mom were holding on by a thread. "Don't you think it's time you two got some rest? Go home and sleep and enjoy your dreams. Mom you stay home in the morning and sleep in, Bob will you please pick me up by ten? They both giggled at me. "Aren't you the patient here?" Mom said. "Yes, that is true but in order to take care of me you need to rest up for when I get home tomorrow." She was happy with that notion and her and Bob decided to leave. "Sleep tight honey" and Bob kissed me goodnight. "I will have pleasant dreams this time." I watched them leave and sipped some water hoping to get good night's sleep after I washed up for bed. That didn't come as easily as I hoped. The entire night was filled with vivid dreams again. I decided it was the medicine and would try to sleep every time I woke up. It didn't happen so easily; I lay there for an hour at a time and would drift off again. The hall noises bothered me, I could hear the nurses in their station, the man up the hall crying out swear words from his head injury and the others crying out for help. I didn't realize how dismal that floor was, so many people in pain. Maybe a walk would make me tired again so I decided to ascent up the hall. I walked very slowly looking as I could without being obvious at the other patients. Sorrow gripped in my heart for them, that they didn't know the relief of being without pain yet and the fears that they had to overcome. One man saw me and I smiled at him and just kept on walking wondering if I should stop and chat with him to try to ease his sorrow. I turned and went back to my room; crawled into bed and thought of these people I had just seen. At the same time when I was feeling sorry for them I was realizing just how lucky I was and that I had made it past that pain. We all did, Bob, Dana, Aja and my mother. I smiled to myself and could not get it off of my mind how bad the ordeal I had been through was, but relished on how well it turned out for me. Shortly after I finally fell asleep again and the nurses woke me up in the morning.

I was going home day! I was so excited to be able to be released early. Only four days in the hospital after major surgery on my brain. It seemed unbelievable. Remember, one of those days I was in surgery for over 10 hours and in ICU for 8. The IV's were disconnected after only one day. I was walking less than 24 hours after surgery. Completely amazing to think that in such a short time I was given my life back. I can go on to see my children and most importantly continue being a wife to my husband. The courage that was needed to drum up to go through this had become a reality. The excitement that bubbled inside of me was overwhelming. The hairs on my arms literally stood up because it was such a feeling that the energy had to be let out. This was all before breakfast. I went into the bathroom and washed my face and brushed my teeth. I remember watching myself spit and thinking how I almost lost the simple pleasure of cleaning myself up ever again. I gingerly washed my face afraid I could hurt my stitches and looked at the bruised woman looking back at me. For the first time after this whole ordeal I actually smiled back at myself. I looked into my own blue eyes and noticed they were aglow with pleasure as well as satisfaction. That woman you are looking at almost died four short days ago came to my mind. I said out loud, "Cheryl, you have made it this far and you will make it through the rest of your recovery." When I smiled the first time I never noticed the smile was crooked until that moment. My face didn't want to work on the left side from the extensive work they had done. The muscles were badly bruised in my left cheek. Then it hit me, I lost some of the muscle there because the tumor penetrated my cheek. I stood back a minute and tried to make the muscles work and there was no way they were ready to cooperate. I concentrated so hard to make a full smile come and I just couldn't. I tried to move the muscles in my forehead. No, they didn't want to work either. I couldn't lift my eyebrows; it was a prominent facial characteristic of mine. It was like I had botox, no movement, no wrinkles, and no expression there. This seemed like an important question to ask Dr. Meyer when he came to check on me later in the morning. Somehow this was important but not enough so that I felt disturbed by it. Deep inside I felt like something was accomplished, and it was, my life was saved and I wouldn't have to leave behind a husband that would mourn and have to figure out a way to survive without a wife anymore. My children could have a mother there for them and some days in the future become a grandmother to help guide their children. This is my new life.

I strolled back out to the bed and sat there a minute. My mind began to wander. What would Bob have done if I didn't survive this ordeal? Would he find someone new to love so he wouldn't be alone? Would he have been simply glad we had our love and leave it at that? How long would he have had to mourn? The very thought made me shudder. The whole idea that I could have left him because of an early death seemed horrible. Would he think of the fun things we could have done, would he feel guilt for the bad times we had to endure that actually made us stronger as a couple? How long would it be for him to laugh again had I died on the operating table? I thought of his warm smile and thought how horrible it would have been if I had taken that away from him. I reflected on how I would have felt had he been in the same situation that I had just put him through. I ached inside my heart for making him suffer with me. Then I turned my thoughts on how for the rest of my life I would dedicate myself on trying to stop the pain for him and do everything in my power to make him happy when we were together. From this day forward, Cheryl Saler, you will do all that you can to bring that man just as much joy in return for what he has done for you.

Then I thought of Dana & Aja. I couldn't imagine going through that knowing my mother was in the balance of life and death. The guilt overwhelmed me again on how I had hurt them so badly inside. I remember how awful it was to watch my father after his stroke and then it became the last time I got to kiss him and let him know that I loved him and hated to say goodbye. It was a very real possibility that they would have to mourn a mother who they knew loved them more than her own life and will always feel that way. I sat and remembered each daughter and the growth stages from birth until now. They made me the proudest mother who walked on this earth. Both of them are caring and beautiful girls, literally beautiful. Not just those faces that are filled with beauty but the eyes that shine beauty from inside. They both wear their heart on their sleeves, so to speak, and that made me the most proud of them. There will never be a person that will walk across their paths and they will never be confused about these people because you will always know what they think. To think I scared the daylights out of them. What would they have done without me around? Would they mourn, would they continue their lives knowing that I felt this way about them? How long would it take after the mourning for the anger to go away that they were only in their early twenties and I couldn't be there ever again? What kind of torture is that to do to your child? No matter if you have a close relationship with your mother or not, how horrible can it be to not have one?

Then I started to dwell on my own mother. How crushing could it be to know you spent those years raising your child and lose that child to something so hideous? To out survive your child would be a terrible thing to do. How crushing could it be for a parent to watch your child go through this even though that person is an adult with grown children? Would she be there for my girls or suffer on her own? It horrified me to think how badly I hurt my mother. I could put it in place because I am a mother too. I felt terrible my father wasn't here to help her through this, I felt terrible I didn't have my father here to help me either.

My eyes welled up, how horrible it was for me to put my family through this. The people I love the most, who suffered because of me. This mess was my entire fault. No, my body defied us. I spent my life eating healthy, thinking healthy, exercising and trying to keep myself a complete person so that I can do things for the people I love. There has never been a greater joy to me than seeing these people smile and enjoy what they are doing and sharing it with them. I wiped my eyes dry and tried to shake off the feeling of how I had hurt them.

A very kind nurse came in and checked on me again. She was almost done with her night shift. She sat with me in the evening and talked to me and told me about her life and what she had accomplished. She was a very interesting young lady. When she approached me she handed me another Kleenex and asked what was making me so sad. I began to spill out my thoughts to her and explain how guilty and sad it made me to think that this put such a damper on my family's life and how horrible it was that I had hurt them. I explained all the things I said in the previous paragraphs and how it was such a miracle to me that I could survive and see them continue to grow and share things with them. She gently held my hand for a minute and went silent. "Mrs. Saler, I watched your family the past few days, do you know how much joy you had given to them being able to survive this? Do you realize you have made them very happy people who smile and share with others when they are not next to your bed? You have created people who love to listen to them and be so happy that you're fine; you have created those around you to feel joy and love for life. This is a special gift that was shared by you, and taught by you. When I met you and started talking to you I was feeling down and upset that things were not going in the direction I desired, you showed me that it really is and told me to stop suppressing my happiness. Do you remember telling me that? I went home and told my family about you, my fiancé also, that you told me to enjoy every day and sadness is deep inside that hides happy and happy is so much better. You said that your father used to sing 'Smile when your heart is breaking' because the good feelings will surpass the bad ones. I tried it and it worked. So while you are thinking those terrible things you are not practicing what you preach, so I made it a point to come see you before you leave. I wanted to tell you thank you. This depression you are feeling is temporary, a part of healing and you are going to heal. I feel it." Her whole lesson that was sent my way definitely made me feel humble and very happy at the same time. I somehow managed to help just one more person in my life path and it was very gratifying.

It was time to head out and take walks for me again. I asked her to let me walk her to the station so she could finish her shift. I thanked her for being so kind and attentive. She hugged me and went into the nurse's station and began to finish her work for the day. From there I made my way up the hall again, walking so confidently, I am going home today, I am going to finish living my life. The elevator dinged and some people with flowers walked out for a loved one. I smiled curtly as best I could, this time it hurt my face a little. The doors closed on the elevator and I watched them walk up the hall, discussing how they wanted so badly for that person to make it through this ordeal. I stood there for a minute and looked at the elevator doors and decided it was time for me to go on my own to the lower floors. Alone, without assistance, by myself, no one to guide me on the way but get to a new level. The doors opened on the elevator and I pushed for the basement level. That terrible level that I feared I would die on. I stepped off of the elevator and walked near the waiting room for families. For a few minutes I watched them holding hands and encouraging each other. I thought about my own family doing that a few days prior. This was never a place I had seen when I was in-surgery and felt so sorry for those people. It was a Saturday morning and they had to be at the hospital when surgeons don't normally work so something horrible was happing. One person looked up at me and I could see the horror in their eyes looking at a bandaged and bruised head. It seemed like a good time for me to continue walking.

I didn't make it very far from there. I stumbled across the chapel and it was barren. I walked slowing inside looking at the statue of Jesus on the cross. For a few minutes I just stood there, looking at the statue.

Thinking of how I stared at one like it in England when I was going to lose my father, how I was praying that the stroke would take him and not let him suffer and how we didn't want to be the people who had to decide if he should be on permanent life support. Then I sat down on one of the benches. For a long time I pondered as to what would be the right words in my prayer to say thank you. How could I say this correctly to my Lord? Before I knew it I started to talk silently there not caring if anyone was listening. "How can I express the thanks that I feel for letting me stay on Earth and letting me finish living? Thank you is such a simple phrase for the wonderful things you have given me. I prayed so hard that you would let me remain here, and promised that I would try to be a better person. You let me stay; you let me keep a marriage, motherhood and family. That is all that I asked for. I understand I have a long road to travel to become well again. I pray that you will help me to achieve this. I pray you will give me strength to help my family understand healing will be a long process and that they will be patient with me. I pray and give thanks and hope that some day I can take this bad experience and use it to help another person. I hope you hear my prayer and understand just how grateful I am. One day I will be able to tell you this in person. Amen." I sat a few minutes there and felt sudden warmth fill me. It wasn't the sun shining; the basement is dark. With that I felt confident my prayer was heard, for another minute I sat until the warm feeling disappeared. Shortly after that I said, "Please lord, will you tell my fathers I miss them, you met them, my birth father and my father-in-law. The impressionable men that passed through my life."

I sat a moment longer and thought about my two dads. I wished my own father had been there and then realized that he would not have handled this situation very well. He loved me with all of his heart and to see me suffer would have been hard for him. Wait a minute; he did see me suffer from above. He came to me in the dream and said he would give me strength. I could feel his presence as I sat there. I relished in the thought to know that he wanted to be there with me. My father-in-law always had a quiet strength that sat with you. A person never knew until you were with him how much power he could have on a person. His unprofessed knowledge was shared in subtle ways with a very kind way, with few spoken words. He never let you go around a bush; so to speak, he gave you any information or advice when you asked for it directly and to the point. Ray gave back more than you could ever give to him. My two dads, why did you have to leave me within a few months of each other? I sat a few minutes more and thought of them each. My father, a hotheaded person who would do anything in the world that you would ask for. I was the last of his five children. The most independent child he had: as well as the one person who would really listen to him on his calls on Monday nights. My father-in-law who tried so hard to give advice only when asked and the only man I ever knew other than his son who would just sit with me in silence or chat about things that were on my mind and never, ever, think that my thought process was out of line, crazy, or insensitive. I sat and remembered special moments with both fathers and decided I was a fortunate person to have known them. That special warmth I felt sitting there with knowing they knew I was thinking of them stayed with me for a very long time afterwards.

It was time to go back to my room. I ventured up the hall. I stood another moment by the family room and tried to reflect how my family must have felt a few days ago. The wave of guilt of what I had put them through came again. How horrible was it for them? It felt so awful to put my husband, children, mother and brother through that. And Diana too, she was so young to have gone through so much in a short life. That young lady had felt so many terrible pains that could make her skeptical of everyone. My heart ached for her. She didn't get the things that my children did. A complete family like we had, a father and a mother who stood behind her together. They did their best as a separated family but she did miss out on the family dinners, someone there when she had gotten home. I then turned my thoughts on my own two daughters. It was so nice that we did that; we shared our days and feelings about the day. We (Bob and I) made it a point to make sure we each had 15 minutes at the dinner table to talk about our day. I stood there and thought about how it was so wonderful that we had held a family together for so many years. A feeling of pride came across me, Bob and I had done it, raised two people that we were proud of. I wondered about how hard it was for my family. I felt a great remorse for them. It was terrible for them to have to face and I hated being the person that had done that to them. I wondered if they knew how hard the fight was for me to get to where I was. To be able to see the smiling faces back at me. I don't know if that would be a realization for them. I looked back at that room with an earnest thought, and a new confidence. I will live my life; I will from this day forward let my family know how much they mean to me.

After that I went back to the elevator. Floor 5. A place now that is going to become a memory. This was a floor that gave me my life to live again. It was a place I wanted to escape and return to my life and it let me, a floor with the tender care of so many people that wanted me to go on with my life. I felt so much gratitude. All at the same time it was a relief that these people were going to let me leave. It was a new feeling that I had never known. I wondered if the nurses felt that way. My life venture was now mine. In a few short hours I would be home. Home, a place I wondered if I would see it again. Home, it sounded so nice. I could go rest there and continue to heal. I can be me again. No person, no outside forces were going to touch me there. It felt so nice I was going there again.

I made sure that all of my bags were packed correctly. Everything was ready for me to return to the place that I love. Our house. A place that Bob and I worked so hard to get. My doggies were there, my things, my home. Like Dorothy said in "Wizard of Oz," there is no place like home. The very thought of going back to where I felt so much fear and thought I would never see again. I was going home today.

Soon after the doctors came to my room with the discharge papers. As I was signing them Bob walked into the room. He looked over the papers and read what he was to do when he was in charge of taking care of me. My mother and children weren't with him. He gleamed with spirit. He was so excited we were going home. He was hiding something and I tried to get him to tell me. It was fine he didn't want to, I left it that way. His eyes glowed and that was just fine with me. He grabbed my little bag and loaded the flowers in the car while I listened to what the doctors wanted me to do when I got home. I really didn't think it was a problem, even though the cautions were great. I had to watch for any signs of dizziness, I had warnings that I could blow my nose and see a little blood and I was not to worry, it was my sinuses and brain healing. If it were a major bleed then I would have to call immediately. I would also have to notice if there were any other symptoms. Any symptoms would warrant a call to the doctors. This was fine with me, I would be vary careful.

Bob came back to the room ready for me to leave. He read over the papers and understood it all. It was such a lot for him to take care of, me. I watched his excited eyes that he got to take me home. He read everything carefully and made sure he knew all of the symptoms to look for. Any dizziness, fatigue, disorientation, and seizures he was to watch and report immediately. It all sounded overwhelming to listen to. Bob with complete confidence knew it was time for him to take care of me. He glistened even with what he had to do. It was completely comforting to know all he wanted was to let me go home with him and become "us" again.

The papers were signed and it was time to go. I walked faster than ever to get out of there. I was going to be free. We had to stop at the pharmacy. It seemed to take forever. I wanted to leave. I sat there on the bench as Bob asked. I watched him try to give the pharmacist the directions of my prescription. I watched him feel just as antsy. He wanted to leave just as much as I did. At the same time Bob wanted me to have the correct prescription for my pain I was about to endure when I got home. Finally they came back to the window. They gave Bob the instructions. I smiled at him when he replied, "I will make sure she is doing well. It's too important to me that she can do this." With that knowledge, my fight was his too. I held his hand and looked into his eyes, I hurt, and this was more than a wife should have to inflict on a husband. My guilt was again surpassing me. Looking at this man I adored it seemed as though it was unfair to him. It was painful to watch him be burdened with taking care of me.

We walked into the parking lot and Bob asked if it was too hard for me to walk to the car. I wanted to. I wanted to make it to my car. I wanted to get to that Volkswagen that I had dreamt of and achieved.

My black VW Jetta. It was filled with all of the flowers and well-wishers' flowers. It was my car that I wanted for a long time. In days gone by I used to look at that make of car and wish that I could own one. It became a reality. Bob opened the door for me and let me crawl in. I sat there a minute and noticed he made sure it was spotless for me. I looked at the back seat and it was so nicely packed for me to take all of my things home. After that I put the seat into reclined and let myself relax and enjoy the ride. I watched Bob drive the car: I watched the road. I was so happy to feel this moment. The man I love driving my car to make sure I can go home and occasionally touching my knee while I rested my sore head. The trust that was there was more profound than any of our days past. I put my head back for a minute and closed my eyes. I relished in the thought of how lucky I was, to know that I really did know love.

We passed by the twin towers as I called it. We passed all of the places I thought I would never see again. It was so delightful. I wanted to close my eyes and rest but the excitement was too much to let me do so. I looked over at this man that made me feel so comfortable and secure. He didn't notice me smiling at him because he wanted to make sure we made it home. Our home. He had things up his sleeve. His smile told me so. After all this time we had been together somehow I knew.

Finally we got to our driveway. I saw that Aja's car was there. When I walked into the house I saw the banners. "Welcome home Mom." It felt so nice and such a relief. I was home. My puppies greeted me with such care and tenderness. There was my family: Waiting and wanting for me to be there again. Angel and Winston were so gentle and considerate. Like they knew they could not jump on me. I bent down and petted them each and gave them a kiss. At the door there were my puppies. My dogs were waiting for me. It was absolutely perfect. My mother stood there with the girls. My welcome was more than I had expected. When I looked down to the recreation room I saw two new recliners. One for the other and me to rest in was for Bob to watch me: or whoever decided to be there to make sure there weren't any wants or needs that was necessary for my recovery. It was a perfect set up. Just for me. My eyes melted. It was time for me to get to the new set in the family room and enjoy the perfect rest area. It became disappointing. I quickly relaxed and fell asleep in my new recliner. About an hour later I felt so much better and woke up to chatter in the kitchen, a chatter I had tried so hard to hear again and felt bad that I fell asleep and missed. I was home, a place that I wished to return to. My head hurt, I wanted so badly to be here again, my home and felt so bad because sleep hit me hard. It really wasn't so bad after all. In the end it was my family that wanted me there and I wanted to be there. The excitement to get back home was completed. I sat in my new chair and listened to my family in the kitchen. They were saying how it must have been a hard transition for me, and wondered if I felt afraid to be away from doctors and nurses. I quietly crept up the stairs at that point and replied, "No, I am more comfortable here, can't you tell by the nap?" They all turned and giggled at me. Those smiles made my whole day again. I had made it back home. It wasn't the building, it wasn't the furniture but it certainly was the ability to come back to the people I adored most in my life.

"Now I get to make a few demands here!" I chided. "I'm getting hungry and hopefully there is a little soup around here for me." I have never seen my family get up so fast to get something for me to eat. Bob had me sit in the chair and put the television on for me in the kitchen. I reached over and turned it off. Mom made lunch for us all and the girls helped her. She made sandwiches for everyone to go with the soup. It was like being a child again with my mother waiting on me. I watched her just like I did when I was a little girl. Dana and Aja helped dish up soup and we all sat for lunch. That sandwich looked so good and wanted that while the soup cooled. I went to take a bite and my mouth just didn't want to cooperate. It doesn't open wide enough anymore. I had to work on half very slowly. For once I ate slower than Dana! After half the sandwich it became too much effort to try anymore and I knew the soup was ready for me by now. I gave the other half of the sandwich to Bob. It startled them I gave up on half of the sandwich and had to explain it hurt too much to chew and open my mouth that far. Immediately Aja was ready to get a knife and cut it up in small pieces for me and I declined. The soup was nice and warming and I sipped that and enjoyed it. After that we enjoyed a cup of tea and chatted a little more. I started to yawn and feel dizzy tired again and excused myself from the kitchen and went upstairs to nap. My mother followed me to make sure I was warm and shortly after Bob and the girls came in the room. They had so nicely gotten me a lift for the bed so that my head could stay elevated. Each of them gave me a kiss and left with the door closed behind them. I looked around the bedroom and smiled at the familiar belongings, cuddled my pink pig and fell asleep.

It was already dark when I woke up again. I stumbled into the bathroom and washed my face again. That woman staring back at me was bruised and sore. My head began to pound and I held the rail down the stairs. It was quiet and both Bob and my mother decided to go to the family room and keep things quiet. Mom was reading and Bob was working on the Internet looking at things. I held the rail and made myself down the next flight of stairs and went directly to my new chair. Bob checked on me and got the ice pack and the next dose of pain medication. I just sat and stared at the tv waiting for the pain to ease. The ice felt so nice on the burning on my head. As I sat there Bob and Mom told me they sent the girls home and that they would call later to check up on me. I was happy to hear that, they must have been exhausted too from all of the turmoil we had been through the past few days. I wanted to sit quietly for the rest of that day. That was soon to be interrupted by family members calling to check on me. It was wonderful to know they cared but I couldn't talk very long. It hurt my head and I would soon turn the phone over to my husband or my mother. It was just fine to hear their rendition of the day and the past few days. It helped them to vent off the many feelings they had.

Soon after supper we went right back to the family room. Bob lit a fire in the fireplace and I sat there and looked back and forth to the fire and television. It was going to be a blur for a few days and that was fine with me. My chair and I were going to become good friends. It kept my head elevated so that I could doze off when I needed and everything I wanted was close by; my husband, my mother and my dogs. If I needed anything all I had to do was ask. This was the perfect place to be.

7.
Recovery

The first full day home was Sunday November 3, 2002. I rested for most of the morning. My mother made our ritual Sunday brunch when she returned home from church. Bob and I spent the morning while she was gone reading the paper and just relaxing. I had the dogs taking turns sitting in my lap. It had been such a good night sleep the evening before that I felt better than I had in days. That wasn't saying much, since it was only 5 days since the surgery. The girls came up for an hour or so in the afternoon to check on me and we visited for a little bit. The boys came with them so the house filled up quickly. It got harder and harder to concentrate on all of the conversations going on around me so I would try focus on one at a time. It was like a stereo was on loud and trying to hear over the music. This time the clutter of noises rang in my head and they just could not be sorted out correctly. When they boys spoke it was easier to hear the lower tones. It was frustrating, I used to be able to pick up on many conversations at once and today I had a hard time concentrating on one. At that point I decided to speak when spoken to and let my family go about the chatter they wanted to partake in amongst them. The chatter started to get annoying so I had to excuse myself for a bit and pretended I had to go the bathroom. I closed the door behind me and just sat there on the edge of the bathtub and tried to clear my head for a little bit. I took a deep breath and convinced myself that I had to go back to the full room of chatter and would then try to listen to just one conversation and answer only to that one, one at a time, one person at a time was all I wanted at that point.

The kids only stayed a couple of hours and by the time they left I was tired again. I tried to creep down to my chair unnoticed and that was not going to happen. Bob checked his watch and gave me another dose of medicine. Shortly after he came downstairs with a fresh fill of ice in the ice pack. I held it to my head and could feel the burning sensation leave. That feeling of the cold ice stopped the pain, the swelling and the constant ache that was prevalent on my head. He put an afghan on my lap, gave me a pillow and went upstairs to help my mother prepare supper. The last I heard was a clatter of pans and the two of them talking about seeing the girls and slumber came to me shortly after that. I don't know how long I was sleeping but it must have been a couple of hours because when I woke up there were wonderful smells coming from the oven that trickled downstairs. I felt a little dazed so sitting quietly was comforting until I could regain my bearings. I heard my mother ask Bob to come wake me for dinner and when he came down the stairs he smiled. "You are awake, are you getting hungry?" "It smells good, guess I should eat a little." As we were approaching the stairs I could hear my mother chopping my food up for me. This sure went beyond any memory for me and she quipped, "Just like when you were little, my little cracked pot nibbling on little bits." You see, when I was only one I had a terrible fall and fractured my skull. My poor parents had to take care of a busy toddler who couldn't sit still. I had to wear a helmet to not bump my head. "We sure didn't think back then I would have a bad head again now did we?" She smiled and got a little teary when she looked at me. "Now mom, both times I am going to heal." I tried to chew on the meat and could only manage a few bites. The potatoes and carrots were soft and didn't need a lot of chewing so that is what I ate. It didn't take much for me to feel satisfied not to mention how it became harder and harder to eat. The muscles were getting tighter as they healed. My cheek hurt where they took out the muscle and felt very tight to move it. I couldn't open my mouth wide enough for a good fork full of food, so I had to nibble like a baby and try not to chew much. It hurt my face and up the side of my skull. The whole left side had a piercing pain when I ate, so it was easier to not chew and slither the nourishment down my throat and into my stomach so that I could heal.

The next few days were resting and talking. Many times I felt rude but excused myself to the bedroom for a nap or to the recliner. I would force myself to walk around between resting so that I could keep my blood flowing. I was terrified of after surgery blood clots. That and aspirin where the only two things I knew would keep those away. Each rest period I felt a little better and would make myself try to pay more attention to the conversations and not fall asleep so quickly. Once I was caught and scolded for not resting more. It was funny to me to hear that from my husband and mother. I would just reply, "Yes dear" and doze off again.

On the Tuesday, 3 days after my release from hospital Kathy came over. She stopped in between studying for her real estate exams. Bob had decided to go back to work and take it slowly for his recovery. He would work half days and get his body used to the task. Kathy and I took a little drive and I snuck into the store and bought myself a pack of cigarettes. She let me have one without scorn and it tasted good. I felt literally naughty for sneaking a pack of cigarettes. For all that I had just survived smoking seemed to be one of the dumbest things I could do. Kathy drove until I finished it and we went back to the house before my mother would become worried. We sat and chatted a little while longer and she had to go home and study some more. She had the state exams to take yet. Remembering how hard it was for the Insurance exams that I had taken years ago I tried to encourage her to go study some more. She did say it was hard to do all that learning a new career and balancing a family. To listen to her it was a familiar memory. It was so nice of her to come and make sure things were going well. I felt so bad because when she had her surgery I was nowhere to be found. Back at that time I had just lost my father and she understood that I had to be with my family then. After she left both my mother and I decided to take a nap in each recliner until Bob came home. As I watched my mother drift off a pang of guilt came over me. How could I do this to her, how could I hurt her so badly and would I ever be able to thank her for being there for me?

Bob came home and was tired from working just a half-day. It had been a month since his surgery and he needed to try getting back into his job. He was tired and glad my mother was there to help. Mom made dinner for us and then made us relax afterwards while she cleaned the kitchen. Bob filled me in on his day at work and how it felt nice to be able to go out and talk to people again. He said his boss dropped by and was startled he was there. Even though it made him tired and ready to come home earlier than he did he wanted to keep trying. It was nice to hear about something new for a change. People who were going on with their lives and talking about what they were doing, including Bob.

The next day while Bob was gone my mother and I headed out to the store to pick up a gift for my brother Paul and his daughter Diana. They had a birthday coming and I wanted to have a little dinner for them and celebrate their birthdays. It felt so nice to venture out of the house and go to a store. Mom stayed right behind me and we picked out something nice for Paul and Diana. After that we headed out to the grocery store and picked up the things need for the dinner and went home. It was a lot of work to get through the second half of the grocery store so when we returned home it was nap time again for me. I began to feel my life was nothing but one big nap but knew that was the way to let my body heal. When I would sleep I would dream of things that I wished I could be doing again and all of the things that could be looked forward to once the healing process was over.

Thursday evening, not even one week out of the hospital we had a little birthday party at my house. Paul and Diana were both surprised to hear I had already ventured out to the stores and shopped for them. My mother and I had fun wrapping presents and getting the dinner ready. Paul and Diana enjoyed opening presents we had given to them. This was something I never thought I could do so soon after surgery and was even stunned how nice it felt to start to be mobile again. They both left early, they had to get up early for school and for work the next day. Bob and I were also tired and he also had to get up early in the morning. It wasn't much past nine and we all were asleep.

The next morning it was time to return to Dr. Meyer's office to get my staples out. Oh how I dreaded that. Every time I had staples out before it stung. My mother drove me to the office and we waited for what seemed the whole day. Finally it was my turn to go into the office. He checked my motor skills again checked the scar and decided the staples were more than ready to come out. Some started to grow into the skin. Those were the ones that hurt and bled a little when he popped them out with his little staple remover. He blotted my head and said I could finally take a shower as long as I dabbed the wound carefully and only rinsed it because soap would sting. I could wash the back of my head with shampoo where the hair remained. The whole front of my head was shaved and by now it had started to become stubble up there. I put my bandana back on and doctor warned me to let it air for a few days when I was at home. No more bandages on my head. If I needed them it would only be when I went out so that no dust would blow into the shuttered area and not get it dirty. Dr. Meyer gave my mother a few instructions and said he didn't need to see me for another month. I could begin to drive again in a week. That felt like freedom, driving my own car. We informed the doctor that I was only taking Advil and not using the prescription medication. Bob was so afraid that I would become addicted to the painkillers and I let Dr. Meyer know that. He smiled and said he rather doubted that would happen to me but understood how my husband felt. Dr. Meyer has the warmest and most sincere smile that I had seen in a long time, it made it so I believed him.

We headed out to the reception desk to make an appointment for a month later. There was one open in 3 weeks or 5 weeks. I opted for the three-week appointment and hoped that my health would be good enough to return to work by then. My mother's eyes glittered with excitement when she heard about my progress. I thought to myself that was one person that I really worried about with my being so ill. She is a strong person emotionally and physically but it still upset me to know that I had put my mother through such an ordeal. We walked out of the waiting room and into the long hallway. As usual we had to stop by the ladies room and off to the parking ramp to the car we went. Mom was worried all of the walking was making me tired. "Oh no, Mom, I feel like I am walking on cloud nine today. It has been such a hard time for all of us and it is such a relief to know I am progressing so well." She grabbed my hand and held on tightly, "Cheryl, I am so proud of you, it has been so hard for you and you just keep on smiling at us to reassure us how well you are doing. I am so happy that you have made it this far and will continue to heal. My prayers were answered." Her hazel eyes got a little teary as she looked at me, "Momma, you have to drive me home for a nap, dry those eyes and smile back at me!" She giggled at my comment; "You didn't change a bit with that titanium in your little head!" By that point in the conversation we had reached the car and searched our wallets for cash to pay for the parking.

Mom headed up to the freeway for our trip home. I looked at the buildings again, the two that looked like the twin towers had the sun shining on them and the silver shaded windows were bright. I remarked on how they looked like the twin towers in New York that had been blown up but much smaller. We discussed how terrible that was for all of the families that had to go through such a nightmare. Mom chuckled at me, "Honey, you just survived your own nightmare." "Oh but Mum, I didn't die. I am not handicapped, so far as we know yet, and if I don't have a seizure in the next three months I am in the clear. Or if my mother doesn't slow down to a decent speed and we don't crash that will be another miracle." My mother laughed out loud at that. "I have driven you around for years before you grew up and moved out of the house, don't you think I am going to take care of my cargo? You just said something that disturbed me, about that seizure possibility. Does that frighten you?" I sat silently for a minute. My mother probed that question again. "Yes, it does in a way, can I admit I am going to set my mind to not do that? If I can pull this off, to not have a seizure, I will have yet another thing to be grateful for. If I can come out of this without any handicaps because it is so early in the game, I will be eternally grateful. Yes mother, these things enter my mind, I read the emails from my online friends that I have gotten recently. They all have so many things that they endured. I understand it upsets you and Bob that I go in the internet and read about other people's brain tumors, but what neither one of you hear is how much support they have given me and have showed me the way of how to fight to become a whole person again, plus some titanium and some screws that currently hold my head together." My mother went quiet again for a minute. "I know you just heard a mouthful of things that run through my mind when I am sitting silently and you think that I am napping." My mother responded, "I knew you weren't just reveling in the moment, no one would after all of this. I didn't know that you were praying not to have a seizure; I didn't know that you understood so much of what was happening. That was a silly statement, I did know that you were researching for information and preparing yourself what could happen. You tried to inform us but we wouldn't listen. We didn't want to know that you could have physical problems forever." We were getting to our exit to West Bend and I was getting tired from the outing as well as the discussion. Not the fact that my mother was listening to how I was feeling, but that I was feeling rather doomed. I could feel myself slipping into self-pity again. "Mom, can we take up this conversation another time? I can't think of these sad things for a while, my mindset is going in the wrong direction and I need to think of happy things for now." She smiled and told me she understood.

When we got home the dogs greeted us with their wagging stubs. We woke Bob up from a nap. Poor guy, this was so tiring for him, not to mention he too was healing from a surgery. I went to him in the recliner and gave him a kiss on the forehead. My mother put the kettle on for some tea. As she clinked the dishes upstairs I checked on my husband and apologized to him for waking him up. He looked up at me and smiled, "No bandages honey. Did it hurt you? What did Dr. Meyer say?" I leaned over to him a gave him a big hug, "So far I am doing well, actually better than that. According to Dr. Meyer, all of my motor skills are fine and it hurt like the dickens when the staples came out. It stings; and some of them started to bleed. In fact it was a little past time to get the staples out because my skin started to grow over a couple of them so it was difficult to get those out. I counted 56 staples across my head, not too sure if that was right. I'm told as I continue to heal the skin will level out. That's a good thing because I don't really want this lumpy thing by my ear. I'm told my hair will cover the scar but forever I will be making sure it will be covered." As I was rambling on I noticed Bob was sitting patiently and smiling at me. "What's the matter?" I asked. "You. You're so cute when you ramble and get excited and it's been a while." Bob always had a way of saying so much in a simple sentence. I couldn't help myself; I just had to kiss him.

"Tea's ready!" we heard from my mother from upstairs. Bob and I walked up the stairs holding hands. My mother smiled at both of us. We sat at the kitchen table as my mother filled Bob in as to what happened at the clinic. Bob kept on glancing at me and smiling as my mother told the story of how I passed all of the physical tests and only "ouched" once at the staples. She told him of how every time the staple remover went to my head I closed my eyes and squinted. Bob listened intently to my mother and smiled at her and then again at me. "I wish I would have been there." I reached over to his hand, "You were there, in my heart." My mother piped up then, "That is something that I believe, she talks about you all of the time. Dr. Meyer wondered where you were and Cheryl filled him in that you were tired from your surgery and she asked you to rest this time. That was the first that he had heard of your surgery. How is your back doing, Bob?" That made him smile. "I am doing very well thanks, it doesn't hurt like it used to and I will add a thank you for taking such good care of us Mom. Before I forget to say it I thought I had better put that in this conversation." My mother beamed, we could both see she knew that we really did appreciate all of her help.

It was getting towards my naptime. I wasn't hungry yet but my mother decided I should have some soup. I sipped it slowly and tried so hard to open my mouth a little more to get in me quicker. After that I put the tray aside and Mom took it up to the kitchen and began to clear up the dishes. I could hear the dishes going into the dishwasher as I began to drift off. I could hear Bob and my mother talking and finally fell asleep. I think I could hear them talking but will never be sure. I thought I knew the conversation but again that won't be clear, ever. I think I heard my mother telling Bob about the physical exam and about the staples and how the scar will eventually even out so that it won't be so noticeable. As I was drifting off I think I heard my mother explaining to Bob that we will have to watch and make sure there are no seizures. I also think I heard her tell him that I was determined that this was not going to happen to me. I also think I heard them discuss that I was not out of the woods yet and that they were going to stay positive in front of me and not let me believe anything else was going to go astray for me. They thought I was sleeping; I was only half way there. It hurt deep inside. My heart hurt, again. I wanted to cry out and tell them not to be so fearful anymore. All I could do was to listen. I wanted to. I needed to plan on how I would help them through this. With that I did fall into a deep dream. It was very vivid, I was standing in front of them explaining how I researched this whole thing. The tumor, the after effects and how much I didn't want this to happen to "us." I vowed in that dream to not be a burden. My families will some day look at me and they will say, "She actually did it. She made it through this ordeal." There will be a day we can look back and wonder how. I will know and wonder if there will be a possibility that I can explain my way up the traveled road my life gave me.

The telephone rang and woke me up. It was Dana wondering how the visit went with the doctor. I could hear Bob explaining his version. As I sat there with my eyes closed pretending to be asleep as I listened in. He sounded so excited that my reports were good. Then he hung up and the phone rang again. This time it was Aja. Again I heard the story. This time I was awake and did listen in a little more intently. My mother noticed I was actually listening. I sat there with a smile as I heard my husband inform our daughters about the progress. I listened to them inquire about him and his recovery. It was so nice to know they didn't forget how their father was recuperating. I reveled in that thought, that my husband and children had such a nice relationship. It suddenly became a pride. My heart suddenly felt like it had swollen like the "Grinch" who stole Christmas. I closed my eyes and envisioned the silly show. I smiled to myself at the silly thought. Then it became a reality. The mere thought that I could remember things from the past. How I can remember when Bob and I sat with the girls and watched these shows and giggle and try to copy the voices. My mind tuned out of the conversation. I decided it was time to work on my memory process. I could remember! I could bring back things from the past that gave me pleasure! The memories of sitting with the children when they were so young, from babies to adults were flooding through my mind. It was like a revelation to me. I jumped up and ran over to hug my mother. She was startled at my reaction. "Mum, I can remember! I can do this, my brains still works!" I was elated. This was one of the things that I was most afraid of. My mother was stunned to say the least. " Did you doubt it?" she replied. "Yes, I was so afraid I could not remember, I knew there was a driving force for me and I was afraid I would not remember why. I know I held on for Bob and the girls, I was frightened. The fear just left me!" I wanted to jump but knew that would hurt, I wanted to cry with joy, but didn't want to alarm anyone. I managed to keep my eyes dry this time.

Bob came downstairs and saw the big smile on my face, even though it hurt. The surgical area was still sore and only half of my face showed emotion. You see the work they had done had frozen half of my face. Those muscles didn't want to work. I couldn't lift my eyebrow, which is a classic symbol of my expressions and only half of my smile worked so it was crooked. He could see that something big had happened to me. I explained to him that the precious memories didn't leave me. I tried to explain how it was so nice to just remember. He held me tightly. It was like he knew just how I felt. He started to shake a little. "Honey, it's ok, I'm working my way back to you." Then he kissed my forehead, " I knew you were going to. I didn't doubt for a minute that you would let us go. Uh oh, did I hurt you're head?" I just gazed back at him, "No, you would never hurt me and you can kiss my booboos away as often as you like." Suddenly I felt very self-conscious. He actually kissed my head for the first time. That swollen, sore, black and blue head that I was nursing back to health. It stunned me. I pulled back. "What's the matter?" he asked. "Nothing, honey. You kissed my head, my ugly head."

"It's not ugly, it's sore maybe, it's yours, mine, ours," he replied.

"Don't fight me honey, ok. We are in this together, remember?" I looked back at those beautiful caring eyes. "Never, I promise." Promises aren't something I will ever take lightly.

That Sunday my sister and brother-in-law came to watch the game with us. Jenny gave me a book and Eddy kept on asking me if I needed to rest. Mom made dinners and helped us all out. Then mom decided to go home for the day. She left quickly and informed us that she would be back on Tuesday. Jenny was surprised and we let her go have some time she needed. I gave her a big hug and thanked her. After that we sat and talked for the evening about the whole event. I could tell by Ed's questions how interested he was and felt bad for not being at the hospital. I reassured my sister and brother-in-law that they were more important now than then. We talked for several hours and at nine in the evening they decided to head home. It was so nice to feel close to my sister again. I always liked Ed. That is why as soon as I heard he was getting a divorce I made sure my sister knew. It happened when a birthday was coming and I informed Jenny. From there a new romance began from an old one and they fell in love again and decided that life together would be good. It makes me feel good to see both of them happy together, and sharing the things that matter most in life.

That evening we lay in bed and talked about the day. Bob remarked how soon it was for me to have visitors and cook for them. I didn't have to cook very much, Jenny brought trays for us to nibble on and we enjoyed the day. Bob did all of the clearing up of the dishes as usual and let me relax and enjoy our visit with Jen and Ed. I thanked him for his help and gave him a hug. Then I explained it was so much easier for me at this time to listen to just a couple of people and not a room full. It was very hard in the hospital, the voices swam in my head and concentrating on the conversation that was directed at me was difficult. Toning out conversations around me was very hard, I wanted to hear part of them and couldn't like I used to. I wanted to be able to answer things said and couldn't make out the complete sentences that were said around me like I could before. I had to concentrate on Bob's face and hope that some day I would have that talent again. As hard as I tried to explain this it just couldn't become a clear version of how it was to Bob. This was something I had to think about how to explain and now wasn't the time.

During the week there were several occurrences. Kathy came to visit me again and took me for a ride. It felt so nice to be out of the house even though I was wearing my cap and no one could see in the van that I was feeling insecure about showing my head that day. The bruising had really settled in so my face had turned purple and green on the whole left side. It felt nice to talk to someone who had been through a similar situation. I apologized to Kathy; I had no idea what she had been through. Amazing how two people could be friends for so many years, go through a similar situation and understand how each person felt. She reminded me that was when my father had just died and I had other things to take care of at home with the girls and Bob. We lived in our little house in Hortonville, our first house that we owned. She had to leave after an hour visit because her boys were due home from school and she needed to be there for them.

A couple days later I had another appointment with my Ophthalmologist. They tested the line up of my eyes on my face and put drops in my left eye to see if the vein in the back was starting to turn red again and give my eye a good blood supply. It had not changed since the surgery but it was explained to my mother and myself that it would take time to heal as the vein was choked for so many years from the tumor that we didn't know about until it affected the sight. My vision turned out much better than expected, 20/40 in that eye. Considering how I had lost the vision and how much damage was done this was indeed a miracle. Again I had to have a peripheral vision test on that eye. There is no pain involved during the test; the pain comes from straining the eye trying to see the little dots in the big circle. For hours after the test my eye hurts in the socket itself. The news was the same as before surgery but it also was early to tell if I would get that vision back. When I got out to the waiting room my mother was sitting there hoping to hear good news again. The eye vision was good so far and more time was needed to determine how far the vision would improve. I needed to make another appointment in another month to check on the progress. I didn't tell my mother it may look like I am peering under water for the rest of my life from that damage that was done. At this point it was most satisfying the eye was healing well and so were the vessels in the eye socket. To me it was satisfying to know that I could keep my own eye and that some sight had come back was more than we had expected going into surgery. Just a couple weeks ago my prognosis was to face losing the eye and disability, worse yet, an early death. My life had been saved and so far that was much more than a person could ask for knowing what a brain tumor can do.

That afternoon some very dear friends from my past decided to pay me a visit. These gals had been close friends since we were 8 years old. We had kept in touch through the years with marriages and children. These friendships were over 30 years old. I tried so hard to hear about their lives and not to dwell on my own. One of my friends, Shelly said that I look really cute in a turban. She always made silly jokes and we laugh so hard when we are together. We sound like young schoolgirls and it feels so good inside. My mother thought that the girls were rather funny too. She giggled with the rest of us. As usual Lynn saw my mother's side of the story and listened intently as she relayed what happened. Lynn and Shelly peered at me the whole time. I could tell they were thinking very hard and trying to understand how it must have felt. That's the caring people they are, always trying to help each other and make each other feel better about bad situations. As soon as my mother seemed satisfied with relaying the information I started to joke around with my friends and my mother. "Look at this, can't rid of me that easily!" I tapped my head and showed them where the titanium was and let them feel the screws that were there. You could feel them through the swelling. "Some day my face will be normal again and you will all have to watch out again, I will give you a complete smile and use the expressions that used to be a part of my character." Shelly laughed. "Look out ladies, she's going to come back at us twofold! Better make fun of her now so that she can get us!" My mother touched my arm and smiled. "She will have the better of us in the long run, wait and see, and worse yet, she is going to be better than ever." I was surprised to hear my mother say that. "You're right, I am going to be better than ever, a better person." Lynn and Shelly began to clap their hands, so did my mom. Lynn shouted out in laughter, "You're right Phyllis, we do have a problem on our hands, that girl that gave us a run for money is going to be more of a challenge." "Stop it, I will never change towards any one of you and you know that!" I retorted. Shelly stopped grinning, "We do, we came to support you honey, we are so happy to see you have come this far. Now show me your house!" Shelly always had a way to divert the subject. I showed the girls our house. We had a little more chat time, and then it was time for them to head back north. It was great to see them but the day made me tired and I really needed to rest for a bit. My mother worked on cleaning the kitchen and I quickly drifted off into my chair. When I woke up she was sleeping in the other recliner. It had been a very tough day on her too, let alone the past week.

The next day it was my payday from work. I asked my mother to take me there so that I could see all of my coworkers. They were so surprised to see me walk in the door. The reception was wonderful. Imagine, one week after surgery and I was walking around like nothing had happened. The only way anyone could tell was the cap on my head and how my mother held my elbow in case I slipped. I asked the receptionist Donna not to let Diane know that I was there so that I could walk back to her work area and surprise her. Donna had also been a friend who helped me in the beginning stages of learning about this tumor. She had her daughter-in-law make the most beautiful silk flower arrangement for me as a gift when I was sick and I thanked her for it. Donna is one of the most beautiful and caring people you want to cross your path in life's journey. Her eyes beam with faith and understanding like an angel. Sometimes when I talked to her it would feel like an angel is answering your questions and giving the right advice. When she hugged me that day I found out about the tumor it was with such complete warmth that a person knew how much she cared.

We walked back by Diane's workstation and she was completely surprised to see me. She jumped up and hugged me. It was so comforting to see her again. I thanked her also for the beautiful flowers that she and Tom had sent to me while I was in the hospital. Diane also called the hospital while I was in there and had Bob call to let the office know how the surgery went. She was the "office crier" and reported on how my recovery rate was doing. It was never anticipated that I would walk in and physically see her so soon. It was "treat day" and everyone asked me to go to the break room and have some snacks and visit with the others in the office. Mary was there and she was completely surprised to see me standing there. She was amazed how the stairs didn't wind me, and quickly got up and served my mother a plate of food. We chatted with several office associates and my mother gave the rendition of my surgery day and how recovery was coming along. It was so much easier for her to tell the story. In retrospect, it was therapeutically beneficial for her. It was helpful for me also, the more I heard the story the more I understood what exactly happened on October 29, 2002.

As we left the office and headed to the car my mother held my elbow to be sure that I didn't slip. She made sure I was safely in the car before we headed home. I told her of all the things on the journey that I looked for as markers on the road. I showed her where that Shetland pony was, where my blue heron friend was on the side of the road. We passed by my brother's old farm and reminisced how my father enjoyed visiting there. We did discuss on how it was so rotten his divorce from Tina was and how he suffered from that. Before we knew it we were home and it was time for my nap. I could feel I needed a rest. This time I went up to our bedroom and slept with the dogs. Winston did his usual sniff around my head to be sure all was well there. It tickled; he was so gentle with me. My dog that was so rough when he played was as gentle as a lamb with me now. He never jumped on me during this time. Angel would come on the bed and sit next to me and whine. When I pet her to let her know it was ok she quickly snuggled in my arms and didn't leave my side. Winston would go to the end of the bed and watch over both of us. If we moved he would grunt and then check on us respectively. First me, sniff around the wound and then sniff Angel and look at her to say, "be gentle." She looked back at him and snuggled in my arms deeper and quickly began to snore. My mother stood in the doorway to see if the dogs were behaving. "It's amazing how they know." I smiled at her and just mumbled, "Night mom, thank you." That day took more out of me than I had thought; three hours went by in that nap.

Before we knew it Saturday was here and Bob was home for the day. Mom catered behind both of us all day. The stress of his own surgery and being back to work was hard for Bob. His back did well during the week but he did tire easily yet. I really didn't help the recovery for him. Mom decided it was time for her to go home the next day so that she can take care of things there. It was past time for her to get some rest and not take care of the two of us. We were so grateful for all that she had done and wanted her to get her rest also. She went to church that Sunday morning and fixed dinner so that we could just heat it up for when Paul came over that evening. When Mom left she hugged us both very tightly and went on her way. She called to let us know she was safely home as we asked her to. Paul enjoyed the dinner and then decided to go home early so that he could be ready for his morning at work. Bob and I were tired too and decided to watch a little television and then get some rest. No, even though we had finally earned an evening alone we did not even consider what most married people would do. It felt wonderful to hold each other in the quiet of the night and talk. We both knew that some day it would be an interest again, for now it was the pure enjoyment of being alone together and holding each other tight knowing what could have happened to each of us in surgery. We checked the alarm was on and soon fell asleep.

The next day was my first day alone since surgery. It felt odd. No one there instructing me, waiting on me or catering to my every need. It had been over a month since I had been alone. I rambled through the house stopping in rooms, thinking deep thoughts. I stood in front of the windows peering outside thinking how lucky I was to see my yard, my neighbors and even the dreary November day that loomed in clouds. I thought about how I almost had all of this taken away from Bob, the girls and me. Most of that day was spent remembering how hard I fought to get to this point. Most of the day was spent trying to think about where I wanted to go from here. Bob called to check on me, both of the girls did too. After I knew that there wouldn't be anymore calls it seemed like a good time to rest. I set the alarm on my cell phone for an hour and a half to be sure that I could wake up and make dinner for a change. This was the first dinner I had made in a very long time. My energy wasn't enough to really do some serious cooking so I settled for putting together a dish to throw in the oven and let it savor. I looked at my oven, my stove and my kitchen. I thought about how hard we worked to redecorate it and how much fun we had doing it. We had all new appliances, new cupboards and new flooring and all of those stencils that I had put on the wall. My teapot collection looked perfect above the cabinets and I just loved the bright yellow. I sat at the table and enjoyed my kitchen, a place where I would get another chance to be able to show my cooking talents. It sounded so nice. One day when my energy comes back....

Bob called again and wanted to know how I was feeling later in the day. He sounded like there was a surprise waiting for me. It wouldn't be until he came home would I know. He came in with a box full of holes and showed me this cute little kitten. He was burned from the car he tried to hide in. His fur was full of oil and he was so tiny for such a terrible thing he just went through. He was a charcoal black-gray. I called him Coal. You could feel when you held him just how afraid he was, the dogs didn't help. Winston wanted to play, Angel never did like kitties and she snarled. Little Coal was so afraid of the two dogs. I took the poor little guy to the basement and gave him food and water. He quickly decided to hide. That is that last we saw of him for two days; he was not litter box trained but he did go next to the box. He hid somewhere that we could not find him but he did come out to eat and drink. We could hear him during the night and the dogs would sniff the basement door that was shut so that they wouldn't hurt him. I talked to both of the girls and asked if they knew anyone that would like a kitty. Aja found someone that wanted to adopt him and she came to get him two days later. He would go to a home that had a puppy to play with and last we heard he was very happy. This was a relief because we did not want to take him to the shelter and risk him being put to sleep. We did learn that the burns to his little head would heal and he would get his fur back. I can understand how no hair on the head can be a little troublesome.

The next few days went without event, which was perfect for us. It had been such a turbulent month we were more than ready for some relax time. Things were actually moving in a whirlwind and we didn't realize it. People were calling the house regarding the progress and we gradually were absorbing the information and what had happened each time we talked to them.

The next week I had a one-month follow up from the surgery with my Neurosurgeon Dr. Meyer. He said all was healing well and that I should be able to go back to work half days the next week. This was exciting, I was able to get back into the world of the living and see my friends. My mother met me at the clinic and was also happy about the news. She treated me to lunch in the café and we went our separate ways. Mom had to go back home because she was so far behind from taking care of us and I needed to go and rest for a while. I tried to nap once I had gotten home but the excitement knowing that it had only been less than a month and able to work again was appealing. I thought of Diane and Donna and how I had missed their company. When Bob came home that evening from work he was happy to know that the recovery was coming along so well and that I was able to go back to work also. He knew I was getting bored with sitting home and felt that I would do me some good to get out again. He was so right.

We celebrated our 26th wedding anniversary that week; it was the day before Thanksgiving. We had a nice quiet dinner I had made and enjoyed the fact we actually could celebrate that many years of marriage. The next day we would spend at my brother's house for the festivities. My family was there and so were some extended relatives of his. They all were happy for us that we were able to enjoy the company. Paul cooked a delicious meal as always and we enjoyed chatting with everyone. The girls came up and Aja made one of her delicious cakes and decorated it beautifully as usual. I was nervous the whole day knowing that the next day I would be visiting an Oncologist. Mom stayed with Paul that night so that she could join us. We went home in the early evening and relaxed until bedtime. It was easy for Bob to sleep; I lay there for hours listening to him in anticipation what the next day would bring.

The appointment with the oncologist, Dr. Schultz was at two in the afternoon. Bob went to work in the morning and came home at one in time for us to get to the hospital. My mother met us there again and we waited a long time to get into one of his rooms. After over an hour a nurse came in and told us the doctor was still going to take a little more time and asked that we be patient. Finally another hour later he entered the room. We looked down at his feet, there was only one shoe on and the other was a hospital slipper. Dr. Schultz examined me and said yes he could do the radiation as Dr. Harris had suggested. He explained the IMRT radiation procedure. He explained there could be some nausea and some hair to fall out again. We were sent home with a book to read about the treatment process. It was completely frightening to read. The whole procedure, the symptoms and thinking about radiation going into my head. We read intently that evening and then I had to put it aside. I just couldn't look at it anymore.

The next day we went out and bought a Christmas tree to decorate and began trying to make the house festive. I sure didn't feel very festive this year. It had been such a shock yesterday and trying to comprehend the whole procedure and wondering if it were really necessary for me to have the radiation. I decided I would talk to Dr. Meyer and Dr. Harris. I needed more of an approval. Bob thought the tree would help my spirits and perhaps it did. He talked of Christmases past and how we enjoyed them with each other and the children. He helped with the decorations and made sure I wasn't making myself too tired. Really it was good that he made me think of something else for a while.

The next evening Aja and Ryan came up for dinner and to help put up the rest of the Christmas decorations. Aja and Dana always loved putting up the tree and remembering times and where we had gotten some of the ornaments. We made it a family tradition when we went on vacations to buy an ornament each place we had been to. This made for conversations regarding all of the trips we had taken and laughing about the funny events at each location. We all laughed and had a fun evening. It felt so good to laugh again. The house looked nice with all of the decorations up again. Maybe Christmas will be good this year. For now the idea of getting ready for the holidays and just enjoying them would be fantastic. We all have come a long way and we need to keep remembering that.

It was time for Aja and Ryan to go home so they could get up early in the morning for week and we had to also. It will be my first day back to work after all of this turmoil. I wasn't sure I was ready but did know I want very badly to share with Diane what had happened. I also wanted to know about my other friends at the office and see how they were. Sure, I did stop in for a visit during my recovery but it wasn't the same. I was going to get back into life, at least part time for now. The slow and steady pace that was my venture had to continue and that was fine. Some day it all would be back in my grasp, work, home, Bob, the girls, my puppies and listening to Norman sing when I arrived home from a day's work. That night I dreamt of how I thought it would be when I returned to the world of the living.

8.
The Real World Returns

For the past month I have listened to the alarm go off and didn't have to worry about getting up. This time I did. Five-thirty in the morning seemed so early again. We lay there for the second alarm but Angel and Winston would not let us sleep any longer. They were hungry and decided to try shaking hands and batting us in the head with the paws would get us up. To save our faces from scratches it was time. The coffee was brewed, set by the timer and the aroma drifted upstairs. We went down to the kitchen gave Angel and Winston breakfast and let them go out. They refused to go outside until we fed them. I poured a cup of coffee for each of us and we sat and watched the news for a little while. We take turns with the shower time and I am usually the first because I take the longest to get ready.

For the first time in a long time Bob packed his own lunch. I took a sandwich bag with pretzels in it to help curb any appetite until I would return home for lunch. After putting my makeup on I carefully placed the bandana on my head and made sure the half bald parts of my head were hidden. Perfect, it just looked like a decoration there and not a concealment of the surgery. The rest of my hair I curled and swooped around the bandana to make it even less obvious. Then rechecked myself in the mirror and the outfit to be sure that everything fit together nicely. Well, almost, there was still a swollen area around my left side of the face. I looked back in the mirror and smiled at myself. "You have come a long way, baby, you're almost there."

Bob was ready to leave by the time I had gotten back to the kitchen. He kissed me good-bye as we always do before either one of us leave. "You look good, have fun today with seeing all of your friends." I kissed him back and replied, "Are you sure, can you tell where my face is still puffy? How's my hair, I don't want anyone to be afraid of seeing my half butch hair cut." Bob gently kissed my bandana, "Honey, no one can tell when looking at you, the brown butterfly decorated bandana goes well with what you are wearing. I really don't think anyone is going to focus on that, they will be happy for you that you made it back." I hugged him "Oh I hope so."

The drive this time was totally different. The horses were outside the barn by the farm. Mr. Heron had left the little pond; it was getting cold, winter is coming. I listened to the stereo as I normally do and enjoyed the ride. My black Jetta and me; enjoying a ride to work and taking in the country scenery. The colors had all left the trees and you could see traces of snow from a few days ago. I looked at my brother's old farm and wished my dad were visiting so I could pop in on him. My father loved to look at the fields and listen to the birds in the trees around the house. I remembered how Paul and his ex-wife lived there with the horses and all of the dogs. That is where Angel came from and remembered how I saw her on the couch in the farm and those big brown eyes loving all of the pets she was getting from me. I fell in love with her the first time I had seen her. Shortly after that meeting my brother had a big bonfire on the property and he enticed us to take Angel home with us. She was a welcome family member, and she knew then to step back because we were losing our Otis. He became old and frail so Angel would help us watch over him. Poor Old Otis, he was the best dog ever, our first Springer spaniel. He was one of the poorest examples of the breed but the best of friends. He and the girls grew up together. I smiled and relished in the thought of how nice it was when he was alive. I didn't see Otis when I was sedated, or anyone else. They all seemed to come visit me before I was to have surgery. My Dad, Dad Saler, Otis and several other meaningful people that passed through my life. Before I knew it I was in Cedarburg and work was around the corner.

My normal parking space was taken so I had to hunt around for another. One thing that was really bad at that place were places to park your vehicle. I took a deep breath and headed towards the door. Inside it still had that musty old bank building smell. I walked up the hall towards my desk. There were a few messages for me in my slot and the light was flashing on my phone. Shortly after that there were people starting to come in for the day. They were all very nice and stopped to say welcome back. Diane and Donna gave me a hug and were glad to see me and many handshakes were given out. Then I began with answering my calls in my messages and there were a few customers that had called to wish me well. I called them and chatted a moment and took care of the policies for them. After that I went through my little stack of written messages to return and talked to all of the customers that needed changes done to their auto policies.

Around ten that morning I was called into a meeting with the two bosses. They began to scold me about things that had been done while I was out. I sat there in awe. How could I have any control of things that happened while I was gone? They talked about a policy that was bound in with my signature. I was never shown the policy to know who it was and decided I had to check into that one. Later I found out that it was signed in my name and it wasn't possible because that date on the policy was one of the days I was in the hospital. They acted like I would remember everything that happened while I was out recovering. It seemed like a dream. How could I know what happened at the office while I wasn't there? No one ever called me or filled me in prior to this meeting. Then I was put on a 6-week probation. None of this seemed realistic. How can someone be called on the carpet for something they had no control over? Who signed the application in my name? Who did these things and why? It was so bewildering and shocking that I just couldn't comprehend all of the things they had said to me. I was so hurt and angry. When those two emotions get together, no matter whom you are or what you have been through are overcoming emotions that make it impossible to think clearly.

That day I left at noon because that was what the doctors had ordered. I was to work half days for a month until I had the approval to return to full time. This was fine as in the insurance world the workflow is slow at that time of year and you end up looking for things to do. When I had gotten home I called Bob to tell him what happened. He couldn't believe it. He did remind me that while I was out sick there was an ad in the paper for my position and that I had called to see if I was to return to work. Legally they couldn't fire me, not from what I had gone through. Mentally my bosses thought that they had taken out my brains with the tumor. It was so humiliating and demeaning to me that the shock didn't leave for days. I couldn't sleep and get my rest that afternoon because I was so upset. One thing I definitely remember, I didn't cry, not one tear. Normally I do when I am really angry and upset. I sat and looked out the front window in my living room and could not believe what had happened. I just stared out the window for hours, petting the dogs and looking at the new snow coming down. When I realized how long I had been basically motionless I went to the window and pressed my forehead on the cold pane. It seemed to bring me back to reality. I just remember feeling the cold and how it relieved the pressure inside my head.

In the morning I had an appointment with the gynecologist for an annual check up. She said that everything looked normal although it seemed as though I was going through the change of life. That wonderful thing that we women get! This doctor started to explain that she would prescribe a hormone to help me along. I disagreed and explained to her that it gave me many problems in the past and that we learned when I had my surgery that the tumor was made of estrogen and progesterone. She pointed out a synthetic solution and began to describe it to me. "Doctor, I don't want to be rude, but the Neurosurgeon told me I would have to go through the change of life all on my own. No hormones, no chances are to be taken. Frankly, after what I went through a few weeks ago, I don't care to take any. My body hormones have to figure this one out for themselves." She smiled, "I understand, we should not take any chances. Now tell me about this surgery." I filled her in, what had happened. She gave me a tetanus shot because it had been ten years and the rest of the information that was needed. If there were any problems I was to call her and let her know about them. This seemed like a mutual decision and I was on my way. Maybe, for just a while I could stop seeing doctors.

The following weekend Bob and I went shopping for presents for the girls and the guys. We wanted to do this early so that we would have time to wrap the presents and not push ourselves too hard. It was so much fun to find things that they needed and to enjoy the time out just being together. Bob decided what to get for the guys and I was in charge of the girls. We never had to think of getting things for boys, let alone men before. It was so much fun thinking about how we would spend Christmas enjoying each other. We had never had the pleasure of thinking about "Boys" for Christmas before. We raised girls.

During this time I did work half days. Each day was spent researching how my bosses had come up with the accusations that were presented to me. Without knowing it they had sent me on a mission to prove my innocence. I researched and found four other applications that were forged with my signature. When I presented them they scoffed at me. I had shown them the dates, they were when I was a patient in the hospital, one was even signed on the day I had surgery! I was appalled, how can I be under sedation in surgery with my head open and a tumor being extracted and have signed an application? How could I tell someone they had coverage when they didn't when I was a patient in ICU? Once I had compiled all of the information they were speechless and still found a way to keep me on probation. They were threatening to take away a status I had worked for three years to obtain. I had to show all of my work to them, all of the quotes before I could talk to a customer to prove that I was able to perform the job. Each day I went into work with a battle, proving my innocence and integrity. After three years of dedicated work and giving them new business worth thousands of dollars, I could not believe that they were disputing what I had done for them. As hard as I tried they would not listen, they actually believed I had wronged the company. If they had really gotten to know me it would have never been a question. If they really had checked the dates when the applications were signed they would have known that I could not possibly be me. It hurt so bad, to have fought so hard to return to the world and to be slammed like a dirty old rug made me feel like a person that had given them nothing, and I knew deep inside that I have given them more than an employee should. Yes, the anger is still there, somewhat, but now I understand. People are afraid of someone who had a brain tumor. They don't understand, I'm not contagious; I checked that immediately to be sure my children would be not affected. My tumor hurt my family and me, not you. You didn't fight like I did; you didn't lie awake at night wondering if you could keep living. You, my former bosses, didn't think of these things like I did. One day you will hurt the same as you impounded onto me, one day you will understand how it is, to know that a battle to survive turned into a fear for the job that you enjoyed.

Just when we thought that all was going well with my health things changed. I talked to all of the doctors to verify that radiation treatment was necessary. We learned during this time that they had to leave a small part of the tumor in the optic area and treat it with radiation. I composed a letter to the Neurosurgeon and asked if this was necessary. The ophthalmologist decided it would be necessary to keep my sight and to let me continue to heal. We learned that if I didn't get the treatments that the tumor could come back and I would need another surgery, like the tumor that almost killed me, the one that took my sight. Could my body withstand that treatment? I didn't know the tumor could grow within six months and take away my sight again and would not be operable so soon. My body just wouldn't be able to handle this nor could they save my eye this time. I was regaining the sight in that eye and I thought that the tumor was gone. Things were not complete, as I had believed; I had to go through more doctors and more treatments to get rid of the demon that was inside my head.

Then came the appointment that I had to see the oncologist and get the mask made. I talked to the doctor and it sounded so scary to hear what could happen to me, again. The whole thing was simply frightening. I was taken to a room and the nurse put me on a table while she heated a plastic thing. Dr. Schultz showed me the MRI scan and how it would be used to measure the points the radiation would hit the optic area. I was strapped to the table as a simulation as to what I was to endure. Then the plastic piece in the sink was ready for the technician to make a mold of my face. It was hot and it instantly made a form of my face. This "Jason" mask was to mark the points that the radiation was to hit me because they could not make marks on my face. They did use a dye to make a point of penetration in the hairline. The temporary tattoo would need to be marked again later when the treatments started. The explanation sounded like I could lose my eye or it would be damaged. It sounded like I could lose some senses that I tried so hard to keep.

I went home and burst into tears. I sat there and waited for Bob to come home. It was all so blurry and confusing. I explained the mask and how I would be twisted and turned on a table, I tried to comprehend the whole thing and I just couldn't. All that became a logical reason to do this disappeared. It just was too much for me to absorb at this time. Bob in his usual way managed to calm me down and decided from now on I should not go alone to these visits until we know further what is going to happen. This was more than a relief. He is always so calming and can listen better than I ever could in a time of trouble. He has the ability to erase emotion and listen to the facts before he reacts. I so needed my "rock" now, his warm loving arms. So many times in our lives I had depended on him and this was needed again. If I didn't have Bob I would never know where to turn and what to believe.

That evening I explained to Bob what I thought I had heard. It sounded like they may destroy the work done on my eye. It sounded as though they needed to kill the remaining part of the tumor but that I would lose sight in the left eye from the radiation treatments. The description of it sounded like it would damage cells that tried so hard to come back and make me whole again. They talked about how the pea size tumor left in my optic area had to be shrunk and how it could grow back in 6 months and undo all of the work that had been done in my surgery. They discussed how dangerous it would be for me to not get enough rest and to get nausea from the treatments. The nurse informed me I could lose my hair again but only in the areas the radiation touched me or passed through me. The staff showed me where they had taken the tumor and all of its octopus feet from my cheek and they had to treat me there too. They informed me all about how the areas that the surgeons had worked on needed to have the radiation treatment because they could not tell if any live cells from the tumor remained.

That was the first day I had coherently seen my MRI after surgery. There was titanium mesh that could be seen, titanium screws that were visible and a hole in my head where the tumor had been. I looked like the bionic woman picture of my head. I questioned if the pressure is now released from the brain in that area would the brain go back to where it belonged. No, it was compressed, for good. It's because that tumor had been there over twenty years and there was now way for it to go back to where it belonged. It seemed amazing to me, to see that I had a "hole" in my brain and skull area and that it would never fill in. That space in my head that would be with me for the rest of my life and never fill in, I imagined it as a canyon that would echo all of the things that I had been through. A deep dark place that will hold every bad memory that was fought to erase but would come back to me when I needed to use them for reference in my future.

Remember, please, they had to replace my skull in the tumor area where that nasty menengioma had invaded; they had to remove some cheek muscle because they found out while they were doing the craniotomy the tumor extended there. The tumor had also extended across my left side of the head and that muscle had to be removed and stretched. The tumor that invaded my eye area was the trickiest. They had to work around the optic nerves to try to keep my sight, my eye. I could have been left with either no sight and an eye or a glass eye. That nasty tumor could have killed me had I had a seizure. That nasty tumor could have killed me if it wasn't discovered. That nasty tumor could have made me disabled, sightless and completely forlorn. That tumor could have made me a dependant for my husband and children that they would never be able to escape. I could have been a burden to my family for the rest of my life. Even though I had signed the papers asking me to be let go if that was the case they would have never been able to do that. My family would want to hold on to me even though I would not have been the person they knew, they would have kept me alive and remembered me and lived with those memories. I thought of how I could have been in a vegetative state in a wheel chair and such a burden on them. I thought of how I could have been blind and have to learn my way around the house. Before surgery I counted the stairs up and down so I would know my way around. When I got up in the night in fear of what was happening to me I would count the steps and practice how I could get around as a blind person. I made sure my silverware was in the correct slots; I remembered the knobs on my new stove so that some day I could cook when needed. I memorized the keypad on my new microwave; I memorized the buttons on the dishwasher. I would stand in the dark and put my finger in the cup as I poured milk into it and then would place the cup in the microwave with my eyes shut. I peeked at the timer after I had set the time for a warm milk to help me sleep. This was just a part of what I went through to think of survival at the other side of surgery had I lost my sight.

Bob patiently listened to me spill all of the thoughts and fears that were presently on my mind and what I had endured. He spilled a little tear and then quickly wiped it away. He patted his knee for me to go sit with him for a hug. As he embraced his arms around me, he confessed he had all the same fears as I had. He held me tighter and said he would not let me go through this alone and wanted more answers to the radiation treatment. He knew my fears had overcome me, and knew that it was time for him to step in again to help me. Again, guilt overcame my heart, it was so wrong that I was putting my husband through this. Again, we agreed to get more information before we told the girls about what was to happen. Again, we had to be parents more than anything to protect our children from hurt. It was horrible to feel these things. Guilt, fear, sorrows, all in one small package that no one ever wants to open, that package should remain on a shelf forever.

That weekend I researched the Brain Tumor society and the treatment I was to endure. I learned so much from my Internet friends. Within a few hours of research my fears subsided a little. Again, Bob was not happy with my searches. He feared I would be more in an agitated state than I was already. When he questioned me I beckoned him to the computer and showed him all about the treatments and how I would be physically. Bob watched a few minutes as I filled him in as to what I had learned and then he just couldn't watch any longer. As I looked up at him I could see he was afraid to know and was wincing about what his wife was about to endure. He was as much afraid for me as I was for myself. As I looked into his deep blue eyes I felt sorrow and shame. Sorry for what I had to continue to put him through and shame for hurting him again.

That Monday I had to call the oncologist and let him know when I wanted to start treatments. I asked that we start after the first of the year and if there was time to wait that long. Yes, it was only three weeks but time was an important issue. It was fine to do so and I was happy with that. We had an appointment to meet with the doctors together on December 16, 2002. I also made appointments for a CT scan, MRI and meet with my neurosurgeon Dr. Meyer. Another full day spent at the Hospital. The patience my husband had was a marvel to me.

That Tuesday I went back to work for a full day. This was a month after surgery. A month after surgery I was back to work half days. It was a long and very hard day. There was a cough overcoming me that was horrible and I felt that way. Because I had just endured that worst possible excuse to feel bad I relented and stayed at work that day. I tried so hard, sucked on cough drops all day long, made a tummy ache from those drops and made it through. It was sheer determination. I was determined to not be sick again. It couldn't happen so soon after such an ordeal. My defenses were down.

The next day we went to see my doctor again. He calmed so many fears that we held on to. He informed us that there was only a 5% risk with the new IMRT radiation treatment they had. He informed us about how he had contacted the medical board about my status of health and how important it was for me to go ahead with the radiation treatments. He informed us that in the end it would be most beneficial for me. Dr. Meyer didn't hesitate to let us know about the risks, as doctors have to and he didn't hesitate to let us know that he would be there all the way to let us know about my progress and how he works with the other doctors through the whole treatment. Those statements made us both feel much better. One thing Dr. Meyer had gained from us was trust and respect. After all, so far he had saved my life, and was working towards my future.

The very next day I just could not take the awful cough anymore and ended up in urgent care. Well, the diagnosis was Bronchitis. This had to be taken care of before radiation and Christmas! I had to be well again. My body just could not handle viruses at this time. I informed the doctor on call what I had just been through and what was in my near future. He sent me home with antibiotics and required bed rest for a day. Just when I thought I was ready to work full time and resume my life again I had to rest again. He chose a medication that would be comparable to what had to be done and to let me kick most of it out within a few days. What a relief! I went home from there, took my meds and quickly fell asleep on the couch with both dogs cuddled up next to me.

That evening was the Christmas party for the agency. The girls went out to dinner and exchanged the final gift from the Secret Santa and exposed whom your secret Santa was. It was a nice dinner and I didn't want to stay late from feeling so crummy from the bronchitis. After dinner and the gift exchange I made a polite goodbye and went home. Bob was glad to see that it was an early night and enjoyed the leftovers that I couldn't eat. We chatted for about an hour and decided tomorrow was another busy day and should let this day finish.

When I had gotten out of work that noon I needed to run to the grocery store to finish getting the supplies for dinner on Saturday. It was already the 21st of December and we decided to have an early Christmas with just the six of us. Every year we try to have a private family day. We raised the girls living far away from the rest of the families and before traveling Bob and I made that tradition. As parents it was much easier than packing all the presents and hauling them off to either parents' houses. When I returned home from the store I made sure all of the gifts were arranged under the tree and proceeded to prepare for the next day. Making as many things as I could for dinner today would make tomorrow easier and let me enjoy the company of the children.

Much anticipation came that morning, waiting and finishing up with the preparations for dinner and making sure the presents were all under the tree and ready for the children, all four of them, both girls and their guys. Everything was in place and for once I was running ahead of schedule. Since I had a couple of hours before anyone would be at the house I set the alarm on my cell phone and asked Bob to make sure I was up in an hour. He did little projects to keep himself busy while I napped. I must have worn myself out a little more than I had anticipated and that hour went very fast. Knowing time was near to celebrate and enjoy Christmas I was eager to get dressed and ready. Shortly after that Aja and Ryan were at the house and then Dana and Chris an hour later. Both girls put the presents under the tree and offered to help in the kitchen. We each had a drink and chatted for a while then ate dinner. During dinner the kids commended me on my fine acting job when I was sick and didn't tell anyone. We all laughed at the funny remarks that I had made during recovery at the hospital. Then they scolded me for the letters. I was waiting for that one to come. I said it was important at that time for them to know what I wanted them to have and they should hold on to them so there won't be any arguments in the future if something should happen. Both girls said they would never destroy the letters, whether or not I had asked them to keep them.

Well, then it was time to exchange gifts. All of them were so thoughtful from the children, all given with love. We laughed and sang Christmas carols in our bad singing voices. Even Angel and Winston got Christmas presents. That kept them busy while we were visiting and enjoying each other's company. I mused at how wonderful it was to be there even with my scruffy head that still bore scarves. The hair had grown to a beautiful butch type cut in the front and I left the back a little longer and curly so that it would appear as though I only had my hair pulled back. We sat in the family by the fireplace and chatted. I noticed Chris was looking rather anxious. Dana whispered to me that he had asked her to marry him but wouldn't tell him yes until he had asked us. Poor guy hemmed and hawed waiting for the right moment.

I went up to the kitchen and Bob followed me to have a cigarette. We never smoke in front of Aja because she hated the smell and complained it hurt her sinuses. As Bob and I were in the kitchen Chris came to join us. We could tell he was working up the nerve for something; well I knew but didn't let on to Bob. Finally he just rushed it out, "Can I marry my best friend?" My husband in his usual manner came back with "Who's that? Hope you're not gay." Chris laughed, "No you nut, your daughter." Bob and I laughed with him and then we knew we had better give the guy a break. Bob said, "Do you're best, we tried for 22 years, now it's in your hands. All you have to do is promise to be good to her." I replied, "That's a very nice way to put it, your best friend, and if that's how you feel and the love trails with it, of course. As Bob said, as long as you take care of my baby you have our blessings." Chris was relieved that was over. Dana came upstairs and looked into Chris' eyes and then pulled out her ring. We all hugged each other and then Dana ran down to show her sister the ring of promise.

That night ended with much excitement for all of us. It was so nice to see my daughter so happy. She and Chris made a nice pair, and I was waiting for the next step. He is very nice and handsome. They both have the same sense of humor and love the same things in life. After the kids left Bob and I discussed the pending marriage. I quipped out to him, "Wow, something I was fighting to live for just over a month ago I am going to see and help plan, our first daughter's wedding." It was such a nice before Christmas evening we spent together. Spending it with my husband and daughters and now we were going to gain a son. Ryan and Aja had a "promise" ring so I guess it was true that our family of two children will be four in the future.

The Sunday after Bob and I spent a nice quiet day together. We were planning the holidays with the rest of the family. This was another nice thought to me, as I didn't think very long ago I would be able to enjoy the holidays. My recovery was coming along well. It seemed nice to think of something else for a while; the upcoming radiation treatments frightened me. There were so many leftovers from the day before we only had to heat them for dinner, which made the day more relaxing for both of us. We both needed some rest before the new workweek and the busy week to come.

Christmas eve I only had to work until noon before we went to Appleton to my niece's house for their celebration. In the morning I was busy taking care of customers and doing my best to complete a day's work in half the time. Suddenly all three of my bosses came to my office and said we were going to have a meeting. They had decided it was a review of my performance in the past year. Fine time to do this, I thought this Christmas Eve day. Well the review went horribly. They decided to put me on probation. The three bosses said there were too many mistakes. They pointed out this was a risk in the insurance world. When I listed what they believed to be things I had done wrong I pointed out how many I could not have made because these things were done while I was out recovering from surgery. The most startling one was an application signed with my name that couldn't be true, the application was signed while I was a patient at the hospital. I pointed these things out, that it wasn't possible for me to do those things if I wasn't there. None of the bosses would listen to reason and believed their decision was correct. I felt completely humiliated and realized that my case could not be argued.

When I got home I burst into tears and told my husband what had happened. He could not believe how cold hearted they were. We both decided that they must have thought they removed my brain and not the tumor. Suddenly I found humor in that thought and started to laugh hysterically. Bob started in too and we decided it was best to not think about this and enjoy Christmas with the families. I would address this work problem when I returned on the 26th of December.

That I did, I provided proof and there was no changing the bosses' minds. They had put an ad in the local paper for my position and when I questioned them about it they said it was not to replace me. I knew better deep down inside. From that day on anger and distaste for a job I had loved for four years overcame me. I called my doctor and asked that he extend my health leave and to keep me on the half-day schedule for a while. He asked what happened and he agreed that I should not put myself under any more pressure and take the time needed. As I went through the office day after day I felt like eyes were piercing through me, they knew what was going on. None of them showed any feelings of guilt knowing that they had put this burden on someone who overcame a brain tumor.

My appointment with the oncologist was on a Friday afternoon. We were to set up the treatments and have a mini counseling as to what was going to happen to me. They explained and showed us charts as to where the treatments would hit my head. A nurse explained how I would again lose my hair. They informed us about the medications that may be needed and that I was to let them know immediately if I became nauseous as it still was dangerous for me to be in a situation where I would vomit. The clinic showed us my treatment room and the monitors that they would use while I received the radiation treatments. Every day for six weeks I would have to get treatments and on every Friday the doctor would have an appointment with me. It was so hard to pay attention to what they were saying because I had been through so much with my health and then with my job. It was like system overload, my mind just couldn't absorb any more for now.

That evening my mother came for the weekend and also my brothers came for dinner. It was nice to try thinking of other things for a while but that just would not happen for me. Finally I told my family what had happened at work and about the treatments I was about to endure. It felt good to let it out and not hide my feelings this time. My family had decided this was not legal for them to demote me for health reasons but proving it would be another challenge. This was not one I wanted to pursue at this time. Maybe after I do some healing and get over the treatments. We were warned I would not have much energy during treatments; radiation also "zaps" your energy.

With the help of my mother we took the decorations down and the house looked bare. It was nice to have that taken care of and not have to do that chore alone. Mom, Bob and I had a nice weekend visiting and chatting about how the ordeal was almost over. One of the ladies came from the Church and brought a gift for me. It was so nice of her and she wanted to see how my recovery was coming along. Mrs. Hatch's husband had been one of the men that gave my blessing before surgery.

Both her and her husband had checked on my recovery from time to time and today she wanted to see for herself how I was doing. It reminded me how nice it was to have so many people care about me.

As I said, the work world turned on me. I spent every day doing my job the best I could and following orders as to what I was to do. I had to show every piece of work that I had done to my boss before I left at noon and he would give me the results the next day on my performance. This carried on for weeks. Each day I was told I had obeyed my orders and each day I left work feeling betrayed and humiliated. There was a manager there who seemed to take delight in my dismay. She had always been very condescending and harsh with her words. It wouldn't faze her to literally yell at someone and she would never show remorse. The whole office would say that was the way she is and accepted it. Not one person stood up to her, until me. I would gently talk her down, like taming a wild horse and walk away. I could feel her eyes like daggers looking at me. If I had not gotten the promotion after the agent I worked for retired I would not have worked for her. I knew she hated that I got the promotion but she was not ready to work full time because she had an adopted son, my children were grown and out of the house so full time work was now an ambition. Each and every day they would give me orders to fill and tried so hard to make me quit working for them. They didn't know nor did I let them know that was my full intention after treatment I would find another job.

New Years was fast approaching. Bob and I have never gone out to the bars or anywhere to celebrate. We have always enjoyed each other's company on this holiday. We make a nice dinner for us and have some shrimp and some kind of dip for a snack later. Years ago we decided since the holidays are so busy we would use this night to make it our own. We would watch movies or the programs that talk about all of the events that happened in the past year. We would also talk about our past years together and then about our New Year's plans. Many times we would put on our old LP's and listen to the music we enjoyed in the '70s and '80s together. We would laugh and giggle about the funny things that those old songs would help us remember. We had shared 26 years of marriage together so there are a lot of fun things to recall. This particular New Years eve we had a lot of feelings about all of the events that happened. We talked about the horrible pain Bob went through when he hurt his back at work, all about his surgery, and of course what happened to me with the tumor and how horrible it was. We also brought out the wonderful things that happened to us that year. How Dana had found the love of her life and wanted to marry Chris. How Aja was so happy with Ryan and they thought of marriage far into the future. How both girls are doing so well and how Aja will graduate from college in June of the New Year. We both strayed away from the conversation of the radiation to come. Tonight we wanted to discuss our accomplishments and the things we were looking forward to.

New Years day is a relax day. We watch football games and sit by the fireplace and just enjoy a day of having to do nothing. I usually indulge in a nap during the afternoon and then work on crosswords or some craft. I've always enjoyed the crossword puzzles. That started many years ago with my father. He would sit and enjoy a pot of tea in the mornings and work on a crossword puzzle. When I would join him we would solve the puzzle together. My dad even had a clue book that would help him. It was very well used; he even wore a hole in the cover of the book from his fingers. If he couldn't complete the crossword he would be dismayed so he used the book for reference so that he could finish it. Crafting became a pleasure of mine too. When the girls were small I would create Barbie clothes for them. We even created a Barbie house and I would make the furniture and help them decorate it. Later I started in with making sweaters in the winter, gloves to keep their little hands warm. Then I graduated to stitching wall hangings and all sorts of things to decorate our homes because we didn't have much money for wall hangings and other things. It was much more cost efficient for me to make the things we needed as well as kept me occupied while Bob watched T.V. I also loved to read books when the children slept or were at school, if I had the time. If you're creative and enjoy trying to be creative it can really fill in for things that people can't afford or don't want to spend the extra money on. Of course there are some projects in the past that didn't work out so well, but at least I tried.

The upcoming week of work I could have done full time but

declined. After all of the events that had happened I decided it would be best for me to just work a half-day. The pressures of what they were expecting of me plus the watchful eyes I had never had before made me feel very uncomfortable. It was like they thought I was going to go crazy on them. This was not just paranoia, it had to do with so many comments that I would get from my old manager and from my bosses. Never before did they ask if I understood something three or four times, never before did they think I needed instructions that many times. We also decided it would be best for me to get as much rest in the afternoons so that my body would be in shape for the radiation treatments that were coming in the next week. All of the warnings were about how I would be so tired and become ill. I wanted to have a week of not feeling exhausted and not ill. This was the first week since my surgery where I didn't feel like sleeping all day. There were many things to study and think about IMRT radiation. Once again I needed to plan how to keep myself as healthy as possible during the treatments and also gain momentum to go through with the treatments. The fear was much like the fear of surgery, except this time something drastic could go wrong from another source. If they accidentally put the radiation beam to my eye it would ruin the sight even more than the damage the tumor has already done. The thought of going to an oncologist's office daily for six weeks was frightening enough. This could also have been a treatment that was unsuccessful. This had to be contemplated also. This machine that was to give me radiation treatment was new to the hospital, it had only been used for a year. The positive side so far in this process is it was a more successful piece of equipment that was used for fine tuning points of radiation.

That week prior I tried to keep myself busy in between researching. I would do some cleaning after I had read information about the treatment. They gave me a manual about the treatment and I think back then I learned it cover to cover. I would sit for hours and talk to Angel and Winston when I was home and go through what I had learned to try memorizing the whole scenario to prepare myself better for my immediate future. Both dogs would sit with their ears perked as I spoke to them. Finally by the end of the week my nerves felt much calmer about the whole situation. I convinced myself I had been extremely lucky because there had never been any disabilities that I had to deal with. I didn't have to learn how to walk again, or use an arm or go through any physical therapy. Another "after tumor" symptom that I didn't have to deal with was being an epileptic. The only things I never did or will escape are the emotional scars that come from surviving such a drastic situation. This scar that extends across my head and the indentation from where my skull was removed and replaced with titanium will never go away, but I am extremely lucky, it could have been so much worse. My MRI's will always show a hole in my head where the tumor was, my brain will stay compressed there, and it will always look like I am part robot on that side of my head. I joke about it now; my files are condensed to one disc instead of 15. My head is stronger on that side because of the titanium. It actually makes a hollow sound if I bonk my head there. You can feel little screws on my forehead. We even laugh about that now, a blonde with space in her head, or a screw loose! I even joke around about my personal face-lift, fewer wrinkles than the average middle-aged woman.

Every day I would try to work on the muscles in my face that were tight from the surgery. For weeks I couldn't open my mouth wide enough for a fork full of food. I ate very tiny bites and chewing was difficult because it made my cheek ache. I was advised to chew gum to make the muscles work harder and make them looser. Then I learned a method to literally expand the muscles. Remember this happened because part of my cheek muscle was removed where the tumor invaded it. I also had to work on the muscles on my forehead. They also became tight after the swelling went down from being stretched back into place from the surgery. Much like a face-lift, I lost almost a half an inch of skin on that side of my head. My face on the left side was like a botox treatment, those muscles didn't move. During the day I would work on lifting my eyebrows so that I could get the wrinkles that belonged on my forehead. It irritated me that the eyebrows wouldn't lift together. Sounds crazy, anyone would be happy to have the wrinkles removed from the forehead, but mine were from smiling and happy expressions, not from frowns. I was always a happy person who saw the best in a bad situation and really was happy in a good situation. To me things happened for a reason, and I did teach my children as they were growing up if there weren't bad times in people's lives they wouldn't know if they were having a good time.

There were also lines on my left side of my mouth to work on. Smile lines there too. I have been graced with them because I created them. To me a middle-aged person who has smile lines is a person who has been content with their lives. I have been so far. I have a good husband, children and have worked to achieve a comfortable life. To me I deserved those lines. It sounds funny to think that someone would want to have lines of age, but when they are swiped away from a surgery and your face can lack character it isn't a funny situation at all. I have always taken pride in the positive attitude that I possess. When I was a child my father used to sing part of a song to me when I was sad, "Smile when your heart is breaking, smile when your heart is aching." The only time in my life that song didn't work was when he died and when I found out I had a brain tumor. Of course there are other times that a person needs to shed a tear to release emotions but shortly after I would do that I would smile and realize things would get better soon. The only thing this middle aged woman wishes she didn't have was the classic red marks on my face from being of British decent and not have so many olive tones to my skin so that I could wear a peach color and not look sick. These are very normal features people don't like about themselves, haven't met a person yet who is completely happy with their appearance, well, women anyway.

I pondered during the week why my employers decided to turn on me. Why did they feel that I wasn't capable to do the job anymore? Did they think because of my brain surgery that I couldn't think or reason anymore? Were they afraid of me? Was it the assumption because I had a brain tumor that I would go crazy? One of my bosses had lost a brother to liver cancer a few months before I was ill, did he think that I would succumb to cancer like his brother? It was a tragic death he had. He went into the emergency room with cramps in his side thinking it was appendicitis and it turned out to be liver cancer and it had attacked his pancreas also. This poor man died within six months and left a young wife and family behind. It would be understandable how he could think that I would have the same thing, gradually fade away. It also was understandable to me how he would feel resentment because I managed to survive. Maybe he felt his brother didn't fight hard enough to live, he could never understand that sometimes fighting doesn't help, when it's our turn to leave earth there is nothing we can do about it. This was something I had to come to a realization with when I was sick, if God decided I had work to do elsewhere I had to do it, or if my work weren't finished here that would have to be his decision. It's wonderful to know he decided I could spend more time with my family.

As you can tell by my writing this book that there are so many emotions that go with what happens when you have and survive a brain tumor. It helped me to relate better what people have to go through with their health. It also gave me more compassion for those who do have to work with disabilities and horrible news of something is wrong with them. It's not to say that wasn't there for me before, it is more intensified now. As a child we would have "Jeannie" stay with us for a week to relieve her parents of the responsibilities that people had with a cerebral palsy child. Jeannie was an adult woman in a wheel chair. When she stayed with us I would take her for long walks around the neighborhood we lived in. One day she laughed and sneezed so hard she threw herself out of her wheelchair. Luck would have it she didn't get hurt but we sure did have a good time with her. This little story was told to you because I was a fortunate child to have parents that believed in teaching me we come in all shapes and sizes and limitations. None of them should ever be used to judge another person, that job is the lord's, not ours.

That whole week in between work and the pending radiation I did a lot of soul searching and thinking about past memories and trying to make sense of this whole situation. I did a lot of discussing these feelings with Bob and he was a good listener to help me resolve things mentally. One thing I am not sure will be resolved is the emotional scars that were made from this. People thinking that I am "marked" or unsure of my emotional state. No, I never contemplated seeing a psychiatrist because I knew these were normal emotions that a person has to go through as a part of recovery. Another reasoning that I had is that people have to work on their emotions no matter what they endure. I didn't feel hopeless or lost during this time period. Those who feel that way, in my opinion, should get help. Being as fortunate as I am, someone listened to me and helped me reason out my feelings. Some unfortunate souls don't get that luxury; those are the people who need to seek out someone who will listen.

By this time in my recovery I was ready for a real hair cut to help me with my appearance. There was minor swelling that remained and I wanted something that would take away from that focal point. I also wanted something that I could deal with and make my hair more manageable when I proceeded on to treatments. Also, from being so ill my hair lacked luster and shine. My daughter Aja had bought me a conditioner and a hair repair kit to help with repairing my hair. So when I came out of the salon that day my hair was cut short on the top and left slightly longer on the back so that if I needed at a later date I could use a "comb over" effect to hide that bald spot I knew was coming my way. If that failed I would resign myself to wearing caps again. Besides, my Jaguar hat was fashionable with my t-shirt to match. In Wisconsin people, men and women wear baseball caps as a fashion statement. Really it was not one I really understood, for a while this would be my fashion. I had several colors of caps, several scarves to wear with my outfits for work and even a turbine looking hat to cover the whole head. If radiation made me lose all of my hair I had the situation covered.

And then it began, treatments, more doctors and more nurses. People, who decided that I should endure this, people who wanted to help me survive. I will never forget them; they will be close to my heart forever.

These people gave me more than I can ever give back to them. I hope they are happy with what they have done, not for me, but for everyone that they help. My medical teams in this process were amazing people; they want to and can leave their jobs every day knowing that they have helped just one person each day. Yes, they also have to face the reality they just can't help someone, but for the rewards of seeing the progress and encouragement they can share are far more rewarding than the negative they have to see. This paragraph is a "Thank you" to them, strong, encouraging people, my husband, my children, my mother and the people who supported me. These people made me want to keep living, even the Brain Tumor Support group I joined. We are Internet friends who support each other, give advice and keep in touch on the progress of how we are doing. That Internet site is still important to me.

9.
Radiation

Walking into that clinic felt very eerie. We scanned the people sitting and waiting for their turns. The clinic staff did their best to try make things comfortable for us all. They had plenty of magazines on all of the tables and pamphlets lined up on the wall in slots of each and every kind of cancer and treatment one could imagine. It was filled with people who did not want to be there, who feared what was happening to them, people in the middle of treatments and knew what was happening. The patients lined up in their chairs and couches, reading, watching TV or gazing into the air thinking about what they were enduring and hoping this would be their cure. The waiting room was gray with purple accents, the usual colors for offices these days. There were three women behind the desk, each performing the tasks at hand. One was checking patients in, letting the nurses and technicians know they had arrived, the other was checking charts to be sure all of the information was correct, the other was off to the side scheduling appointments. My appointments were all scheduled for 3:30 p.m. Monday through Friday. The scheduled times for radiation were all set up weeks ago. Every Friday after treatment I would see my doctor.

We watched a couple of women called in. They were there for treatment for breast cancer. They all had varying degrees of hair loss and you could see they were either beginning treatment by the color they had and the hair that existed or the others had hats and bandannas on or wigs to cover the loss of the hair. They looked weak and tired and almost a yellow color. The breast cancer people had a "group" amongst themselves and would talk about the treatments to each other quietly in one area of the clinic.

Then there were the men; they were getting treated for prostrate cancer. One man looked very sore and tired. Don't know if he was hurting from the recent surgery or if he was actually sore from the treatments. The other men seemed fine and had their wives or family members with them for comfort purposes.

Other women were there for uterine cancer or ovarian cancer. They had symptoms of radical treatment. Chemotherapy and radiation were a part of their lives. Many of the breast cancer women were having the same treatment while others were getting only radiation. You could tell by the looks on their faces as to what treatments they were getting. Someone was nauseous from the treatment and she kept the nurses busy.

I was the only woman having treatment from a brain tumor. There was one man there who was escorted by either his boss or his wife. He was in terrible shape from it all. It was a malignant tumor that he suffered from. He, like myself wore a cap to hide the recent surgery and hair loss. His treatment was more aggressive than mine. His treatment time was before me. He also had to be on the table for half an hour while the radiation hit the parts of his head that needed treatment. That poor man had a malignant tumor. Since the discovery and surgery I had learned that men have a harder time recovering, if they can because most of their tumors are malignant. I watched this poor man daily for three weeks. My husband caught sight of me watching and held my hand. "What are you thinking about?" I just smiled at him and said, "I am wondering who will survive this ordeal the least hurt, who will make it, who between the two of us will they be able to tell that the tumor is a part of your history." When I looked into my husband's eyes I could see his uncertainty was just as deep as mine. Again the pain of what I was doing to him hit me; the pain of what I was fighting for was also hitting my heart very hard. No one had the answers for me, not even a doctor could tell me what I want to know. As I looked at the chairs and people around us I wanted to get up and run away.

My treatment as with everyone who has this happen to them the treatment was different for all of us. I had IMRT radiation. It is a more direct treatment. The radiation has more of a laser point to it that targets only the necessary areas instead of all through the head. This was needed because of the location of where the tumor had remained. Behind my eye, so they needed to target all around the area and not hit the cornea or directly at my eye or it would damage my eye and the fight to save my sight would have been a useless endeavor. My tumor was benign so the treatment could be done at long intervals but with less intensity of the radiation at the points needed. Regardless the treatment had to be done, to remove or shrink the pea-sized tumor that was left behind and to finish killing any cells that were left behind. If those cells would not have been killed a tumor can grow again and it could be malignant this time. It was a necessary treatment that I had to endure. If I had decided against the treatment the tumor in my optical area would grow back and I would need another surgery and they may not be able to save the eye this time. Not a pleasant decision to make, but hope and prayer were my options that this would work.

Bob and I sat there and waited for my turn. Finally they called my name. Bob settled into a cup of coffee and a magazine to wait. He also turned the TV to watch Jeopardy, an intellectual program that was the challenge that people enjoyed. They would ask trivia questions as a challenge to its players. Bob always liked that show because he has a wealth of trivia knowledge locked up in his brain that can amaze anyone how he could know so many answers to the game. We always would tease him about how he knew so much that he should try out for the game and could be a winner too. I turned back to look at him settled in and he smiled back at me to give me reassurance.

The nurse weighed me and showed me the way to my treatment room. There sat a huge machine that had a space ship type part that would move around my head. I was instructed to lie on the table after I removed my bandana. The technician put a pillow under my knees to try relieving any pressure that my back would have. She put a blanket over me and then proceeded to line up my head on the brace for my neck. Then the mask was placed over my face and I was bolted to the table so that my head and neck would not move. The mask had the markings on it for where they were to hit me with the radiation. My partially baldhead had the marker dots for the treatment also. I had a blue dot on my head and a mask on me! The technician tried to make sure I was as comfortable as could be and then left the room. As she exited she closed a huge lead door. I noticed as I walked into the room that door. It seemed at though it was at least a foot thick. Then the machine and table started to make a noise. I tried to close my eyes and relax. The machine would make a whirring sound and the radiation would penetrate my head for ten minutes in that area. Then the bed would move and I would get treated in another area for ten minutes. This was a thirty-minute process and I had to lie there very still and not be able to move as much as an inch. This was the first time in my life that I felt sick being moved around like a slab of meat on a table. I vowed then, no more roller coaters and fair rides that turn me around and upside down.

It seemed like an eternity in there. It seemed like they would never finish. Finally the door opened and then technician came back in the room. She unbolted my head and helped me to sit back up. I felt very dizzy and had to sit a minute before I could get myself off of the table. Finally I made it over to the chair that my things were on and put my scarf back around my head and went out to the waiting room to Bob. He had a challenge going with the other people waiting for their loved ones already! It was nice to see he was filling in the time. I went past the desk after Bob helped me with my coat and the ladies cheerfully said, "See you tomorrow!" I smiled at them and said, "Yes, see you then." As we walked up the hall to the elevator we looked at the horizon of the city. We could see the ballpark and the roof was open. We could see the tall buildings that were only a mile away. It is a nice scenic view actually. Milwaukee is known for the Brewers and Miller Beer. It has a park with garden domes and couple of different colleges. The hospital I was treated at is a Medical College. Every visit and exam there was a doctor learning a practice or an intern working on a doctorate. Finally up the long hall was the elevator. When we got to the bottom floor we had to walk past the pharmacy and the gift shop out to another set of elevators to the parking lot. We usually parked on the third and final floor because there were more empty spaces there and I worshipped seeing the outdoors before and after treatments.

Our drive home was during rush hour and the traffic was thick. Not like Los Angeles or Chicago but enough to have to be careful as to what the other drivers were doing and careful to merge into traffic. Some days were worse than others. Ten miles into the trip we would pass a pair of buildings and we dubbed them as the twin towers. We would talk about how horrible that was for so many people and how life had changed for us all since then. I would mark the trip by streets in one of the cities we had to go through and by the stretch of highway 45 markers. West Bend was 40 minutes from the hospital so there was plenty to look at on the way there and home.

When I got home that day my head felt hot, like it had been burned. I took out the lotion that was given to me made especially for radiation treatments. It felt so good and soothed the spots immediately. I decided it would be a good idea to use it before treatments. I also was terribly thirsty and downed a tall glass of water. Bob and I worked on supper and then decided to relax for the rest of the evening. Angel and Winston were happy, they were fed and ready to sleep on the couch. Winston passed by me and sniffed my head, kissed my cheek and took his place on the couch next to Angel.

For the first week I felt fine, no fatigue or nausea. Not until the first Saturday morning after treatment. I tried to keep myself busy and not think about it and to my dismay that wasn't going to happen. Then I tried to take a nap in the late morning and just couldn't close my eyes because the room would spin and I would feel worse. The nausea was the same as when I was pregnant with the girls. Finally early afternoon I called the hospital and asked what I should do. Crackers didn't help; tea didn't soothe me, nor did 7-up. I could only drink water and then still felt like I had the worst flu ever. The nurse called back and called the pharmacy for some medication. I couldn't drive so I had to wait for Bob to pick it up. The nurse explained it would be dangerous for me to be sick; the pressure on my head would cause problems for the healing and recovery. I felt way too sick, that medicine took about thirty minutes to work and I felt like a new person again. Bob made some soup and I felt much more relaxed and could keep the soup down.

Sunday morning was much better and I wanted to get out and shop or just walk around for a while. We went to Wal-Mart to get supplies for the upcoming week. I was looking at some caps on the rack while Bob went to the photo department. As I rounded the corner I came face to face with a person who was also balding and looking at the caps. We looked at each other and smiled. She was much younger than me and was hoping to find something more fashionable. I asked her if she had seen the caps in the end rack, we could get three for the price of one. I asked her how she was feeling. She told me her energy was running out and it was time to find her family and ask to leave soon. It was her naptime soon and that without it she can't face the rest of the day. Her treatment was chemotherapy and it had been three weeks already, she could feel the strain on her body. I wished her luck and wandered off to find Bob. It was just like walking into and meeting my own ghost. I could see the fear in her eyes, like mine, I could see how tired she was, like I will be later and I could tell she was embarrassed about the hair loss and knew that I was going to feel that way again soon.

The next treatment I wandered out to the waiting room feeling like I was walking on clouds. The room seemed different and my feet were wobbly. My body felt like it was traumatized. As I got to the door of the waiting room, Bob stood up as he saw me coming and grabbed my jacket and helped me put it on. I felt like I was going to pass out and concentrated on walking and looking forward only at my husband for security. We said goodbye to the receptionists and that we would see them again tomorrow. We walked up the long hall to the elevator and went out to the parking ramp to the car. Because I was getting treatments we had gotten stamps so that we didn't have to pay for parking every day. We gave the attendant the ticket with my stamp on it and proceeded to drive back home. I put my head back on the headrest and tried not to be obvious. Whenever I would close my eyes I felt dizzy sick, when I tried to watch the road and the streets and landmarks it made me feel worse, there was no escaping this time.

Half way home Bob finally asked why I was so quiet. I filled him in on the radiation table and how it turned me around so that the radiation could hit the intended spots. I filled him in about the woman I had met. It was such an overwhelming day. It was only a half hour but all the things that happened in that time seemed like I had lived an entire day. I felt the effects of the radiation and knew what was coming my way. We feared what was going to happen together, we discussed it on the rest of the ride. It felt good to express my fears and explain what was going to happen to me. The conversation seemed to help relax me and stop the queasy feelings that were churning within me.

Bob told me about the people he had met while he waited for me. They all decided to have him the personal channel changer on the television so that they could challenge each other for the game show. He informed me he read the magazines and even decided he would go through them and work on the crossword puzzles to pass the time. I listened to him and decided how lucky could a woman be, her husband beside her trying to help her heal. He had been so patient so far and I had to make him go through another bout of illness, mine again. He told me about the different people he had met and how they chatted. I was so happy to hear that he had found a bond with the other families that were waiting for a loved one to heal or conquer the horrible diseases that were in the oncology department.

When we got home we made some soup and settled in for the evening. I worked on my crossword puzzles again and we enjoyed our Monday night programs together. Shortly after we had gotten comfortable the phone began to ring. Each daughter called to see how it went for us at the clinic. My mother phoned after the lines weren't tied up and wanted to know how I had fared the day. I couldn't tell them very much at this point. It could only be said that we had a long way to go before this would be over. This was something that both Bob and I didn't really want to think about, we needed to take one day at a time. Each day would mark another for illness before healing. I knew that deep down inside and never verbally said it. This was to be another road to try very hard to get rid of the demon that lived in my optical area. That little pea size tumor that had to get "zapped" and hopefully it would work and I could be free of this disease, the brain tumor.

Over the passage of that second week I began to feel more and more tired, and each day I tried to hide it and deny that I was feeling that way. It seemed so wrong to feel that way so early in the treatment. By Friday I was completely exhausted and staying awake past 7:30 in the evening became a challenge. Because I didn't want to leave Bob alone to watch television but still I would fall asleep in my recliner. I hated to be alone. I feared that feeling. That was the physical side of the emotions that I felt because really I was alone in this venture. I was the one who had to fight and try to come back to life. I was the person who had to endure the treatments and do all that I could to keep my strength so that my body could endure this. It really doesn't matter if it is chemo or radiation treatments, they both make your body weak and your emotions tired. Every week they weighed on me, and every week I had to have a physical to test my motor skills.

Let me explain that process. Being a Medical College people are trained to look for the finer signs of things that can go wrong. The technicians and my doctor would test my hearing and my balance. Every week I was asked if I had a seizure when I wasn't there. That statement made me start to wonder, if a seizure had come my way, and a person doesn't know what is happening when they have one, how would you know if you did? I asked the nurse that question one day. It seemed like a very logical question to me. She informed me I wouldn't know but that people around me had to notice and they had to report that to me. But, if it had been a small seizure that lasted only seconds would I know it had happened? Would I know that I had lost a minute or less? This was perplexing to me. So I grilled her. If in fact that I had a seizure would I know that I lost that time? Would I be confused after the seizure? How would I know? She said I would know but that I wouldn't know until a later time. If they work like, for instance an

Alzheimer's person, can anyone tell? There was never a clear answer to my questions, only that I would know or the people around me would. So I went on with the tests, walking the straight lines like being tested for drunk driving and checking my balance. Tuners ringing in my ears to see if I could hear them, making me watch fingers as they traveled around my head and defining how many were there in each side view and identifying how which fingers were being held up for me to see. They would look into my eyes with lights that blinded me for a minute and then ask about my eyesight. They would check my reflexes and neck movement. This was a weekly affair. Soon the technician would mark my chart and leave. Dr. Schultz would come in and do the tests again. He would read my chart to be sure everything was entered correctly. On the very first visit I was given the 24-hour line number in case of emergency.

I had officially earned the "green card" at the hospital. The green card was my pass to say I was a patient needing continued care. That thought bothered me. We knew the way around this huge hospital and could give people directions. This huge place knew me by my first name. This is not a good situation to be in. I never wanted any hospital or pharmacy or clinic to call me by my first name without identifying myself. Hundreds of people go by and through this hospital; I could no longer be anonymous. As friendly as they all were and a caring staff that made sure the patients was comfortable, you never want to be known by your first name. That "green card" made me a permanent patient. I will never be able to escape this, not for a very long time.

In only two weeks I was feeling the effects of the radiation treatments. I was tired; I looked pale and green. My skin tones were beginning to change. You could see the burn marks from the radiation. Every day I would look in the mirror and see a woman who was getting broken down. Every day I would also think how I had to overcome this and some day my life would be good again. There will be a day that I will smile back at the reflection and realize that I did overcome this. This was a fine line of hope I held on to. One day I will see the person who had overcome the life threatening disease and be fine. My odds were slim, but each day in that mirror I would tell myself I will be able to have this be a memory and marvel how I managed to overcome this. I would look squarely into my own blue eyes and put sheer determination in them. I would talk to myself at the reflection in the mirror and coax myself to think positive.

Within the third week the symptoms had become worse. Yes I did get up for work and do my job for a half-day. I was washing my hair and a handful of hair came out into my hand. I gingerly stepped out of the shower and patted my hair to stop the dripping. I looked at the towel and there was a huge clump of hair in the towel. I went to the mirror and wiped off the fog and looked at my head. I could see that it was coming out on the top of my head and there was a definite bald spot. After I had dried myself I went downstairs where Bob was watching the news and showed it to him. He held me close. "You knew this was coming." I did, he did, and I was hoping I wouldn't have to go bald again. I just looked at him dry eyed, no words had to be spoken. The hug from him worked just fine.

I put another scarf on my head again. Hiding the falling hair and afraid the scarf would rub more off. I just looked at myself in the mirror and could only sigh. It's something I hoped would be temporary. A woman losing her hair, it's a sign of getting treatment to get rid of a horrible thing that almost killed me. This was getting harder and harder to face. I stood there and started shaking again. Then it was time to quickly turn those emotions off and realize this was something that needed to be done to save my sight and to try not to have another surgery. As hard as this was, I had to do this; there wasn't any option for me. I was stuck in the mode of trying to save my life. This had to be accepted for the time being, there was no choice.

My mother came to our house for a week to help out and let Bob have a week off from going back and forth to the clinic. My daughters took their turns with watching the treatments and to drive me home. They watched what the machines were doing to me during treatment. I never knew until they told me what was happening on the other side of the big lead door. All of the technicians working on me explained it to them. One day I was sitting with my mother and my head got very itchy. I scratched and all of the hair fell out of my head on the left side by my temple. I just looked at it in my hand in shock. I gave the handful of hair to my mother. She smiled at me trying to understand what I was going through. I left the waiting room and walked quietly into the ladies rest room and began to scratch my head so that the pain would go away. My hair fell into the basin and I just stood there a minute and looked at it before I rinsed it down the sink. It was such a horrible feeling. I looked back at my reflection and took off the scarf that was hiding that part of my head that had already gone bald. It was now time to readjust how the scarf was to be worn. As I looked at myself I tried to talk myself into some more courage. I sighed to relieve the fears and sighed again to give myself strength. When I walked back to the waiting room my mother was searching my eyes and looking at me with direct pain in her heart. When I sat next to her she grabbed my hand. "I can and am going to get through this" is all I could whisper, and pulled my hand away from hers, I never looked at her and muttered, "Just stand by me, please."

The next day the technicians gave me an Angel from the cancer society. She was a cute little ceramic trinket. They told me I had earned her because whenever I had treatment I would talk to the other patients in the waiting room and never show fear but give them encouragement that we would make it. I felt honored and humbled. I talked to these people because I wanted them to overcome that cancer they were fighting. I thought they had bigger fish to catch than I did. Some didn't have surgery yet; some were children with parents afraid for their children. To me we were all people who were fighting to become healthy people again. I knew some of us were not going to overcome the fight, but I just couldn't let them give up. Life was something we all had to cling to; love was even greater. I was told that they decided I should have the "Angel." They told me when I walked into the waiting room everyone smiled and were happy to see us. It was never something I intended to receive, that little statue of honor. It was just that people in the room were afraid, just like me, and I didn't want any of us to go out of this world feeling lost or lonely. We were a group that needed each other. Is that something that deserved a token of honor? I didn't feel worthy. It wasn't an honor for me; it was for them, my life has revolved around just one smile to make a person's day worth living made my day feel complete. I started to wonder if I was being selfish. It was important to me to see another person happy, it will always be. When someone is crabby or rude to another person I feel sorry for them and begin to wonder what made them so sad or unhappy that they feel others around them should have to feel that way too. In an "oncologist" setting, we are all sad, we are all fighting for life. We have to create a smile to make it easier. So this "Angel" statue belonged to the clinic and the people there. Not me. Our "Angel" belonged at the reception desk to be shared. I don't know if she is still there.

We met so many people on this venture. One woman who was elderly was having treatments for her uterine cancer. One day while we were talking she was letting me know about her tattoo for the treatments. It totally surprised us when she lifted her shirt and pulled down the front of her pants to show me the marks that were made on her body. I looked in amazement and noticed it was shaped like the state of Texas. I blurted out, "Oh my, you have Texas on your belly!" We all laughed at my comment. From that day forward her husband and daughter thought we were totally entertaining people. The family would talk to us every day and wait for us to get there. This lady waited for me every day and refused to go in for her treatments until she could see me and say something that was important to her. Well, if this gave her hope and the power to keep fighting for her life this was quite a gift I could give to her. I felt honored she felt this way about me and I was honored she wanted to share. Her daughter spoke of how her mom wanted to see me again every evening. She told me how she fought hard to keep her soup in her for strength. Every day this lady told me she was a good girl and ate and felt better later on when she did. I didn't do anything more than tell her what the nurses told me, nor did I ever ask any questions other than how she was feeling and remind her of how important our naps were to get our bodies healthy again. Months after our treatments I got a call at work, her daughter said mother was not doing very well and asked that I call her in the hospital. I did, directly after I talked to the daughter. When she heard me, she called me her English girl. She told me she had had enough, she was tired of feeling sick, she was tired of being tired, she was tired of trying to fight. I asked why she wanted to quit the fight. I wanted a good reason. She couldn't give me one, I asked her to not back down now, and she was past the half way mark of recovery. Before I knew it, I was begging her to keep living and hung up the phone. A few days later the daughter called me at work again, I burst into tears, mom had made it, and mom would not give up the fight. She told her that the English girl called, and that was all she said. I never did hear from them again, to me this is good, that wonderful woman made it. Do I think I saved her? No. She just needed a little encouragement.

Finally on February 14 I finished with my diploma. I didn't have to go back there for six months. I was told my hair "might" grow back. I may have a life of comb-over or I may live with healthy hair again. The doctors would need to check on me every six months with an MRI and show me if the tumor shrank or grew again, I refused to think that way. I made a promise to myself. Secretly and never told a soul, I am going to come out of this nightmare and be a whole person again. I won't be sickly forever. This will be a memory, a lesson. Some day I will be able to look behind and be grateful. There is going to be a day that I will be grateful for making it through this ordeal, grateful for a husband and children that were there for me. We all made it this far; we will keep going forward. We will be thinkers, planners and people who will know that tragedy can be fought and overcome. There will be a day that we can look back at this and smile, and remember there is a god that can help. Ask him. He gave me a job to do, some day I will know what it was.

Other people that were there were not from our society, so to speak, but we found each other. One man had been through so many different cancer treatments and he refused to give up the things that made him sick. He would wander in alone, no family and not a person there to show they cared for him other than the "group." We felt bad how he was a so badly dressed man, shabby and torn clothes. He had a lung cancer that would not cure nor could there be a cure. His days were numbered and he knew it. We never did learn his name, we will never know if he had made the ordeal. My instincts tell me he never did pull through. I remember seeing this poor man who was abandoned to face this alone. He was very gruff and downright crabby. He never smiled; he only talked to the receptionists.

There was also a very young child there; he was no older than ten. He held on to a book every day that was about his treatments and the story was about a dog who had a brain tumor and how the dog went to the machines to get better. He held on to the book very tight every day and read what he could. One day he ended up next to me in the waiting room. I looked over his shoulder at the book. I said to him, "My head hurts too." This little guy looked back and said he was tired and how his head hurt and how the surgery made him hurt. My heart went out to this little guy. His dad held him as he tried to not let him fall asleep before the treatments. The look in his father's eyes had a small glance of hope left. When they ended the treatment the little boy gave me his book. When he asked that I keep the book we read together I asked him if we could leave it for another person to read. He was happy with that thought. And so the book remains there for another child to learn and cope with a brain tumor. Again, we don't know if he survived, we only know when he left the clinic he was ready to go home and finish healing to play soccer with his friends again. He hugged me when he left, I wished him well, and hope he is out on the field having the time of his life, being a boy.

The nurses at this clinic were people that deserve awards. Every time we passed through they wished us all well. I will never understand how they can do this job every day. They know that some people will never make it to the other side of life and do well again. They fight for others to survive and give them strength and hope. These are truly people that need to get rewards. Oftentimes I would wonder why they chose that particular profession. Did they have just one more person they wanted to help? Did they have a loved one go through this ordeal and become more understanding about how it affects people? These people really have the strength and stamina it takes to be a complete human being with a purpose. I can't imagine how rewarding it can feel.

My mask still sits in its bag in the basement. I have pulled it out a couple of times. When I look at it the feelings of fear become an anxiety attack. People don't understand how I could feel when I see it, unless they have done it. It gets better every time I look at it and realize how it had to be. That horrendous feeling of being in an oncology department of a hospital to fight for life, until you get to try it you can't know.

The smells that are there, you can smell machines trying to save a life. You can smell the stench of cancerous tissues that are trying to take life from someone. You see people lined up in a hallway waiting for treatment or recovering from what they just had been treated for. They say that a dead body has the most obnoxious smell that you will ever come across, that it will make you gag. I am not entirely certain about that, don't want to know if it is true, but I can tell you burning rotting skin is not pleasant either. Sick bodies emit an odor that is hard to forget.

When I walked out of the clinic on my graduation day I didn't look back. I think I even made Bob walk fast, and he has twice the length of leg than I do. The hope of having to go there once a year for a check up was what I wanted. Some day, I would dream that they would say they don't want to see me anymore. Every time I have to go back there I feel afraid of having to do this again, grateful I did the unthinkable and have been told I don't have any disabilities other than emotional scars and a horseshoe scar across my head. The face-lift that saved my life, the one you don't want to see or know about. 4 short months ago I was told I would most likely die, most likely have a handicap of some sort to inconvenience my family's life as well as my own.

We walked so fast to the car that day we were both out of breath when we got there. I impatiently waited for the door to open on the passenger side of the car and quickly got in from the cold. Bob just grinned over at me; he didn't need to say anything. Again I got the parking sticker ready as we exited that ramp. This time the drive home I felt like I was free for a while. I didn't have to go back to the clinic for three months. For a little while I could work on gaining my energy back again and start to live my life all over.

A month later the weather started to warm up, one March day it was so beautiful as I drove home from work. The snow was melting and the sun was shining like never before. It was the first time in a long time I needed my sunglasses. I was absorbed in the trip home. The sights of all of the animals that had been let out of the barns again to romp in the fields in the refreshing spring air. I turned up the stereo and opened the sunroof in my Jetta and felt like I was driving on a road to freedom. It was the first time in a while that I had felt this good. As the wind whipped through my hair I took the bandana off of the stubble on my head and let the breeze pass through it. It was such a beautiful feeling that I started to giggle out loud. Then within a minute later I realized I missed my turn toward home and laughed even harder at myself. Me, the spring winds, my little dream car and the freedom to get well again. I yelled out, thank you Lord! In all that time since October I had never felt so happy inside, hopeful for a full recovery.

I went back to the clinic two months after that, with a full head of hair again. The receptionists didn't recognize me at first. I didn't look sick anymore, I had hair and not a scarf. When my nurse came to get me she gave me a huge hug, she held on tight for a minute and then stepped back. "I knew there was a beautiful person in there, you glitter again when you smile, and you don't look ill any longer." I smiled back at her, "Still nervous again, here I am praying Dr. Schultz will give me good news from that MRI." She held my hand, "It's all hopeful for you now." The nurse couldn't tell my anything but from the look on her face I could tell she knew I was on the mend. Dr. Schultz said that there was a little swollen part in the MRI but wasn't sure if it was from the surgery or if the tumor had to continue shrinking. Everything was above target so far and that I didn't have to go back to see him for another six months. When I smiled back at him he said, "That swelling on the outside of your face will gradually go away too. You won't know other than the scar you had surgery there, but from the looks of the MRI and the way your face is shaped now a stranger would even notice there was work done on the left side of your head." I questioned as to when I will be able to take another real bite of food because my cheek muscles were still very tight and I was eating tiny bites at a time, he advised me to chew gum to work the muscles again.

We had appointments every six months for the next year and a half. I had MRI's taken and then finally he said all of the swelling had gone away inside and all that was left was the scar from the surgery. My face had returned to its normal shape. During that time I also had to see Dr. Harris my ophthalmologist every three months. Finally he said that my sight had returned to 20/20 in both eyes. I won't get all of my peripheral vision back but I had gotten used to turning my head. I had to continue to see him and after a while my gland dried out in the left eye. Then came cauterization of the tear ducts to hold the liquid in my eye and that it needed to continue healing. That hurt like the dickens! It doesn't matter if they freeze your eye or not, sticking a needle in the eye socket is a white-knuckle pain. I squeezed that chair so hard I know I left nail marks in it.

For those few months I stayed working at a part time pace until I would not have to go home and take a nap. When they tell you radiation also "zaps" your energy they are not joking. That entire year after surgery was an up and down of energy levels and emotions. Still to this day I need a nap here and there, but only indulge on weekends. Once in a while an emotion or situation will surface those old scary feelings again and I have to quickly remind myself that I did heal.

10.
Life Goes On...Thankfully

Thinking about this whole thing again has been very difficult. But, unlike most of my peers in this world that have gone through this, I am one of the most luckiest people that have had Angels, family and the wonderful lord that kept me going, the things that made me want to keep living. All the things that make a person fight for life.

The most important was, I wanted to continue to be a wife. You see; I love my husband as you can tell by the prior writings of this book. I love my husband more than myself. He has been there for our children and me. He is my goal. I want to be there for him. I want to be the wife he asked to marry many years ago. I have needs that are not met yet as his wife. Bob is the most understanding and kindest man that a person could ask for to be your partner. He has seen me through the worst time of my life and the best. I have done the same for him. We have endured things as a couple that a lot of people don't have to go through. We have survived. I love to be with him, whether he is happy or sad. I apologize to him many times for hurting him so with the death threat that I proposed to him. There was a time I honestly thought that I would have to say "good bye." I asked him to marry and fall in love with someone else if I had died, I asked him to love another and feel happy again.

That sounds funny, I know, but he is such a good person that he needs to share his kindness and love that he can give. I am so lucky to have such a man in my life that can do just that and I was so concerned that he would be lonely that I could not share his wisdom and kindness. I truly felt that someone could be so blessed to understand that, that that person would be able to share that with him. My concern was that a vibrant person should never have to be alone. Bob did divulge to me he didn't want to do that, he wanted to appreciate the love we shared and remember it as we had it.

How could a woman be so blessed? I knew just how lucky I was before surgery and how lucky I would be on the other side. He helped me in so many ways that really I could never really put this into words. We have loved each other for over 25 years, there was a day that when he asked me to marry him I did say, "Do you know what you are saying?" At that time I was only 18, he was 20, did we really know what we were doing? We were young people in love and not really knowing what the road ahead had to send our way. We made it so far; I really don't think we are going to stray form each other.

Many years ago I made promises to our girls. I love them equally and they also have been there for me. Dana and Aja are my shining lights. I promised that I would be there for them for a very long time. This was important to me to fulfill as their mother. I knew before I gave birth to each of them that it would be one of the most important things in this world that I would be a part of. It's a treat to be able to say as a parent that our love is an equal thing, that we can divulge secrets together and all of the happy things that go along with a parental relationship that a mother and her daughters can endure. I have loved them when they are happy and when they are sad; I had tried to guide them to be a happy person, deep inside where it counts. My only wish is that I was able to give them that. We had so much fun together that any bad time was washed over in raising them.

Dana was a child that demanded a lot of attention in her own way. She was content as a small girl but then in school felt very lost and alone. She needed a lot of guidance and never really understood just how wonderful she was. Her talent for putting things on paper and writing her emotions halted her from speaking them for years. Now that she is a grown woman she can do that. She would write for hours and I encouraged her to do so. That way she could work out the feeling that she needed to feel. Dana could create beautiful pieces of artwork as a child and never knew just how impressed I was with her ability to work things out in her mind.

Aja had the ability to say what was on her mind and not mess around with debating it. I was also very proud of her for that ability. If she didn't like what you did or said there was and no argument until you showed her the "other" way of doing things and thinking about others. She could sing like an angel, and she needed her very own special care for a while. We learned that she had Juvenile arthritis, and we worked with her doctors and made her life as comfortable as we could. We bought heating pads and sleeping bags for her, we fought the school system to show that she had a problem moving around from pain, that it never affected her thought process and reason. We, (I) did all of these things for my girls because they deserved it.

After radiation it took a year for my hair to completely get healthy again. I lost half an eyebrow from the radiation treatments. My hair refused to come back there. I used to pride myself in having perfect shaped eyebrows, now they are a little deformed. This is a small price to pay for being able to live. If the hair chooses to come back there or not that is fine. For now I will use a pencil that can conceal it. It seems so ironic to me because I could never figure out why anyone would want to pluck out the eyebrows and then pencil them back in. Now I understand, they just don't want to grow where they belong so then you have to find a matching pencil to your hair color. The challenge will be some day I will have gray in my brows, and will it matter then if my eyebrows aren't a perfect set anymore? After what I have been through it really doesn't matter now. Not everyone is so blessed to have started with good shaped eyebrows. I guess I don't have to be different in that area. I just remember that my grandfather used to love the way they were set on my face and said once that my grandmother had eyebrows like me. I wanted to be able to carry something profound that she had.

Then a while later my teeth started to hurt. I had major damage to a tooth while we were on a trip. It just happened, I was eating a sandwich at a fast food restaurant and it cracked in half while I was chewing dinner. That hurt like a dickens and I couldn't eat the rest of the sandwich. I gave it to Bob to finish. I was nursing that tooth to the max and finally it hit. Then the big crack and then ouch! I had to work on trying to open my mouth wide enough for a dentist to get in there. That is a process, for a full year I could only fit a small electric toothbrush in there without pain in my jaw and cheek. Thanks goodness for Oral B brand toothbrushes. I was always very finicky about my teeth; this was the only toothbrush that I could fit in my mouth. I went on the Internet to my tumor friends and asked them how do I get the muscles in my cheek to loosen up enough so that I could be examined. Many of my cohorts told me that they had a "finger" method. For a month you work on your mouth, first taking two fingers and making the jaw open. It ached, and then after you get past the aching point you put three fingers wide in between your teeth and work on getting your mouth to open that much wider. You have made it when you get to four fingers. That's as far as I had ever gotten. A person should be able to fit your own fist in your mouth with ease and be able to open wide enough for a dentist to get in there to do their work. I can't and won't be able to do that. My mouth is only so big. Then that brings a question to your mind. How did I eat for over a year? Little bites. That simple. One at a time, I have finally gotten to be able to eat a meal in less than a half hour. I asked the doctors and they suggested chewing gum. That works fine when your mouth and jaw doesn't hurt.

That tooth had to say "good-bye"; the radiation and illness took its toll on it. That hurt in a way, other than the physical pain. It hurt because like my eyebrow, I was proud that I had made over forty years with healthy teeth. I decided the consolation prize was that I had survived a brain tumor. When the dentist told me that the tooth had to be extracted and we couldn't save it, while she was apologetic about it, I told her that she could be giving me horrible news like "you have a brain tumor." This was something that I had to expect from radiation and surgery. A week later I was at an oral surgeon getting my tooth extracted. That hurt a lot afterwards, in fact for a couple of weeks. My mouth felt abused, invaded. Not just from the extraction but from having to hold it so wide open that it never had to do since surgery and the last cleaning and x-ray. I couldn't eat or drink for a couple of days. It stung like the dickens. My jaw hurt too, so any chewing was painful. The cheek muscles that had to be removed needed a new stretching and they didn't want to do that. The end result is a space in the back of my mouth. Some day I will be able to afford an implant. No one other than me will know a "fake" tooth is there. Think of it this way, the implants will have screws made of titanium that will match my skull.

The other physical effect I had was my left eye decided to quit making the correct amount of tears. You see; the surgery damaged the gland that makes tears. The radiation also did that to me. The gland was also damaged from the radiation I went to the ophthalmologist for months after the surgery. He had to look at the measurements of my eye and how they were placed on my face. I had eye exams that never could be anticipated. Every time I went there the tests lasted over half an hour to an hour. There were visual exams, checking my face and how the skull was accepting the alignment of my eyes. Let me try to explain.

When you see a specialist he has to make sure that everything is in place. A special ruler comes out to be sure your eyes have gone back to where they belong. Luckily for me it was just one eye. The measurements are charted. Then you have these drops that dilate your pupils. The doctors use machinery that looks very deep into your eye. They needed to see if the vein that fed my eye was doing well. The last time I checked the vein did not want to cooperate and did not get full blood flow, but they weren't too concerned about that since my sight was coming along. Then they put this stuff in my eye that made it turn a florescent yellow to look in with the black light. That gave the progress and current condition of my cornea. It showed any tearing, scratches and recovery stage. My cornea had suffered a lot in the left eye from the radiation. I am told I see 20/20 out of the eye. It's not really what a 20/20 should be, some days it's like looking under water from all of the scratches and damage. If I use the eye drops like I should it is better. When my eye gets dry and scratchy I have become used to putting drops in my eyes. If you ever sat in front of a fan full blast and held your eyes open, that is what it feels like. Or did you ever look into the breeze on a windy day or when you're in your car with the defrosters blowing at your face you might be able to understand how it feels. It hurts, to blink, to look either way, left or right, it feels like your eye is going to be torn apart, the cornea is going to get ripped off and you will never see again. Did you ever look at yourself in a cracked mirror, or a dirty windshield? That is the best description I can give to you. That is the sight I have in my left eye. It works pretty well when I use both eyes. The peripheral vision is there and I can see things coming up on the side of me again from the left eye. You can't sneak up on me anymore from that side. This is good; I can see when I drive from that side. It used to frighten me when that sight was lost. Maybe I have just gotten used to it. Turning my head is automatic now. But I am so grateful I can see three-dimensional that was gone for a very long time. I don't have to look for the lines to know when to step up or watch my bearings.

After many check ups it was decided to cauterize my tear ducts. That really hurt. Not the burning the ducts shut, but it was the shot in the eye. I have grown very used to pain, when someone complains of a minor headache or hangover I can't help but think how they are being big sissies. They never had to survive a lightning bolt headache that screeches through your body and makes you stop any movement. It hurts so bad that you feel sick to your stomach. That was the feeling when they put the needle in my eye to make it numb. This was after they gave me a drop to make the shot itself not hurt so badly. Now the drops for numbing your eyes are something that you may want to know about. It's the strangest feeling. You can feel your eyelids tingle and go with a burning feeling and then it feels like you're not blinking at all. You can see that you are. You can see the moisture being replenished in your eye but you cannot feel it. Like novocaine when your tooth is frozen, Blink, think you have tears, feel the eye move but not. The only way you can tell your eye is moving is by scanning the room. When you scan the room you can see the machines in front of you and the doctors all trying to determine if the job they are working on will do the job that is intended for you.

For two years after the surgery my life was full of doctors working on my sight and my reflexes. It was visit after visit of these things. I had to prove and hope that it worked that my sight was getting better. After a time they all realized that I was going to be as good as they could get it for me. I have learned to look mostly out of my right eye. I have learned to depend on that for the best vision. I am supposed to and do put a night cream in my eye and that helps a great deal. I am supposed to use drops more than I do during the day to stop the dryness. I have grown to knowing when the slight sting comes to immediately put the drops in my eyes, which I do. Things like good sight have become an obsession with me. I get annoyed when my sight becomes blurry. I also get frightened and afraid all over again that something is wrong. Many times I look into the night with the left eye and have come to the understanding that there will never be sight there again in the dark. Shadows and looking for light is no longer a saving hope for me. But then again, my right eye has completely taken over and it compensates. That used to my weak eye. My right eye has become my balance, my focal point. To change your train of thought per eye is a feat, I have managed to do just that.

Other things have happened along this trip too. Until you have done it yourself you will never know what it is like to look in the mirror and appreciate your hair. If your hair bounces, if it doesn't feel or look damaged is really a major thing to some of us. It is a pride thing for women. If you can brush your hair and feel the scratch and pleasure it is a feeling that is taken away and given back. The nerves on my scalp are trying to grow back and it causes extreme itching to this day. When I scratch it feels so good to feel hair there again. But one never scratches too hard because you also know how it feels when you do that hair can fall out. The feeling of looking at my hand or seeing it fall into the sink will never go away. I still have dreams of losing my hair and having to wear a hat or turban on my head to hide the loss of hair. It's also gratifying to have a little wave or curl where the hair fell out. I can now "bounce" my hair with the right cut and make it look decent.

My left eyebrow will never fully come back. Therefore I came upon the understanding why people use pencil. For 45 years I could never understand why women would pluck all of the brows out and then pencil them back in. I used to have perfect shaped brows. Now a pencil helps them look like they have shape. That's a minor thing again. My eyelashes are there and I can still use mascara. I still have my blue eyes. I can hide the missing brow with pencil. Only if I point it out people do they notice.

Another thing, I have an indent in my head and a spot on my forehead that you can see something happened. No one can tell. People will get really funny looks when I let them and show them they can actually touch a spot on my forehead that has a screw poking out. Not only am I blonde, but I also have screws! Now isn't that a topic of discussion? I can really play the part if I so choose. The other factor that I find amazing is that where the tumor was, there will always be a blank area in my MRI scans. Really, there is a space, void, whatever you would like to call it in my head. There is Titanium, some screws and an empty space permanently to be a part of me. I will never forget what it was like to look at the first MRI that showed the tumor there. That scary feeling will never leave. Now those scans look like I am the bionic woman, metal, space. That space holds a lot of things that can never be refilled. That is not as bad as it sounds, that Menengioma won't ever be there again. Like my daughter says, "Meanie menengies, did their mother wrong."

Some more wonderful things happened since then. I have life and can continue to have that. Not so many of us get to do that. We in my "society" of brain tumor survivors have to suffer with disabilities. I was so worried that I would be a burden. Well, here I have sat for hours writing this book and have gone on with my life. Will I ever forget this ordeal? Never. Will I forever be grateful? You really don't need to ask that question. Every day from then on I have done things I never did before. If the sun is shining I bask in it, if it's raining I think of it as moisturizer, when it's overcast, I will look for the cloud shapes and think of how they could become something I never was.

The first event of the summer was that our daughter Aja graduated from college. We were so proud of her. She had made it through hours of study with great grades for a college person. Aja made it to the dream I never had. She worked full time, studied and attended classes as well as had a man fall in love with her. This is something I had always wanted for myself but so happy that my daughter could accomplish knowledge from her books and schooling. I watched her for hours concentrating and trying to learn all that she could. Many times I would marvel how she could sit there and absorb so much. Then she would turn around and go off to work and enjoy her friends and getting a giggle out of life and those around her. We had a big family gathering to celebrate she had done so well. I cooked and cleaned for two days before the party. It felt so good to be able to do that. Yes, it was tiring but then I was given a gift. I conquered the "Obstacle." I was supposed to die, and I got to enjoy watching my child make a huge accomplishment.

Other wonderful things happened since that time too. My daughter fell deeply in love and she married the man that meant so much to her. We had a wonderful time planning and shopping for her wedding. Picking out the bridal gown, choosing the bridesmaid gowns, decorations and guests. We three girls had a wonderful time that was stressful as well trying to get the whole day ahead of us planned. We enjoyed it all. Making the decorations for the reception, picking out the jewelry and veil, what the girls would wear and what I would wear as mother of the bride. The men had it easy; they could wear a tux and be done with it.

Our shopping day finding a bridal gown was comical as well as wonderful. We went to a lot of bridal shops and finally found the perfect dress to go on my perfect child. I chocked back tears as I saw her standing there. It was so hard to believe my first-born daughter was getting married. The tears were never from sadness in any way. We looked forward to the day where she would be happy beyond belief and the day was near. We spent another whole day shopping for the bridesmaid's gowns, and I totally enjoyed being with the girls. I relished in past memories of how I enjoyed being involved in the activities at school and being so proud of my girls. As a mother when they were young it was an honor that they asked me to be involved with their lives. I still feel that way, and all through both of their lives I never want to get in their way.

Dana shopped and did price comparisons for the decorations for the wedding. She found the best way was to make the decorations and it saved a lot of money. We had so much fun with the stupid glue gun and sitting around the table laughing about how clumsy we could be. The decorations turned out just as Dana hoped. We three girls spent time together again laughing and giggling about silly and stupid things. It was wonderful.

After gown fittings and jitters galore we finally made it to the wedding weekend. The rehearsal went well and we all felt the next day would go well. All the music was chosen, the musicians were ready, the DJ was ready and we decorated the hall after the church rehearsal. Then we were all ready for the next day after a long night making sure the hall would look nice. We had a lot of help from family members and friends.

The big morning came. We girls left early to get some coffee and get our hair done for the special day. We went out for lunch and completely enjoyed ourselves for the last time that Dana would carry the family name. We were on the road to get back to the apartment and the hotel when we hit a traffic jam. We sat there for over an hour and Dana was beginning to panic. Aja was teasing about my little car and how we should just bypass traffic and after a few tears from the bride to be I decided that was enough and we were getting dangerously close to getting to the church on time. I turned my little Mini Cooper and went around the traffic to take an alternate route to get us all to our designated places before it was time to head off to the church.

We all made it on time. I busied myself with helping Dana and Aja get ready. My girls; my bride my maid of honor, my children, in a state that only a mother could dream of. I stood there and looked at both of them all dressed so pretty and looking like women now. It was breathtaking. Bob wandered downstairs to see where his girls were and I could see the look in his eye on how proud he was of them. Pictures were taken of us getting ready and then it was time to get upstairs and start the wedding. I kissed both girls on the cheek and told them just how beautiful they were.

Dana stood at the top of the aisle waiting for her turn. I was led to the front as most mothers are. Dana turned to her father as I was getting escorted and gave him the $2 bill he had given to her as a child. "Dad, you told me that on my wedding day I was to give this back to you." He was amazed that she remembered and found that bill. I knew what she had planned. Bob held on to that bill until after the wedding. It now goes to her child when he or she gets married. Bob and Dana marched to the front of the church, we gave our daughter away to a man we hoped would love and cherish her forever. Chris welled up in tears and continued to do so through the wedding. We all had a hard time looking at him; I had to stop when I wanted to cry.

The day was wonderful; we had relatives come from England and from miles around. We didn't have much chance to sit because there were so many people there that were happy to see the kids. That day will forever be an impression in my mind, my beautiful girls, my husband and the family and friends that wanted to share the day with us.

These were the things that I had fought so hard to stay on earth for. If it was to be decided I should have died that day when the tumor was taken I was satisfied to know I had made 45 years of life and a marriage that most people dream of and children that make parents proud. But that didn't happen; I am still here and enjoying it.

I left the job that demoted me after I became ill. It hurt what they had done to me and I just couldn't trust them again. Every day that I went to work I felt under scrutiny, they watched everything that I did and made notes about how they felt I was crazy or "missing" some brains. They would take paperwork that I had done and not let me read it and make accusations hoping that I would slip up. I would insist on reading it and then defend myself but it was never good enough for them. They wanted me out of the business and set me up to do so.

I found a job at another insurance agency and that man decided that I was nothing but a scapegoat. He had some bad business before I was there and it ended up to be my intentions to destroy him, or so he made it out to be. I had customers that had claims and falsified their statements as to what was written on the insurance policies. Being the person who wrote the policies it was my fault. He also had a wife and child that didn't like me being there. After he bought the condo in Hawaii and spent thousands of dollars on his motorcycles, second house and children in college he decided that he should fire me on false accusations. My firing came the week after I refused to let him kiss me, after I told him that my name wasn't "Sunshine" and I would prefer he used my correct name. I lost the battle for unemployment; we lived a full 5 months on one income. It hurt us financially as well as emotionally.

It seemed like it was a bad dream for a full year, recuperating, getting over the emotional scars that the tumor left as well as the physical scars. I felt completely doomed. I wanted to scream and tell the world that life is not over when you survive a brain tumor. This is why I wrote this book. The fight and the struggles are something I wouldn't wish on my worst enemy. People who know me understand what it was like. Others don't want to know. I don't tell anyone unless something comes up that it is deemed they should know.

How do you think I dealt with this? When someone says it's too hot or too cold outside I don't look at life that way. Sure I feel the heat and cold. I look at it as another day I get to live. Strangers think I'm silly when I say to them how it's another day we get to live and enjoy.

I think of disabled people in a different way now. It's a fact that I could have been one of those people, I smile at them and remember how lucky I truly am, and my compassion to live has been enhanced. I remember very clearly going out into public wearing a scarf and hat full of bruises and not having any hair on the front of my head. People do stare, it's out of disbelief, it's out of shock and they don't understand. I won't ever ask them to understand, just believe it when someone says they know what you are suffering with, we understand. Our scars are hidden, but they cut very deep. We brain tumor survivors will smile at you with the most caring smile you will ever see. We will never want to compete with you; we just want to help you. We will listen no matter what your woe is; we will guide you if we can. If you need a soft shoulder or a reason to battle for what you want, that shoulder is there.

In my passage this past couple of years I have seen children trying to survive from some sort of cancer. I have seen the elderly fight for life that may only last a couple of years. I have seen men fight prostrate cancer, others heart problems, women fight breast cancer. We managed to keep fighting, and will continue to do so. It's a funny thing, but if you think life is worth keeping you will fight for it. Not just for your family, but for yourself because you want to be there with them.

As you see this book was not all doom and gloom. I hope I showed at least one person that if you want it bad enough you could accomplish what you want. Maybe someone out there is feeling lethargic and feels that hope is gone, maybe someone needs to know that it is all worth the trouble that you have to go through to succeed.

I don't work in the insurance business anymore. I grew tired of the misplaced competition. People who will think nothing of walking on you just to get ahead, these are people I don't want to be with anymore. Since that time I turned down management positions, I am no better than the other person I work with, I respect them and I want to be an equal. I don't want to ever leave my place of work again hoping I was fair or made a decision that was good for all. I choose to not work overtime anymore because I want to go home and enjoy life there. My life, husband, children and pets are my priority. If I feel I want to nap, I take one, if I get frustrated that my house is dirty I clean it, if I want to sit on my bed and pet my dogs I do just that. If you think you don't like me, I don't care anymore, how you want to feel is your decision.

Life became something more and new. I never gave up being grateful before I was sick, now I am even more so. If you can get up in the morning and enjoy the day in front of you, this is an accomplishment. When you look at the world and want to change a negative attitude keep in mind it isn't you, it's them. You can't change them, don't try, smile and remember just how horrible it is when you think the world hates you and you hate it. To me it's such a sad situation to have worked yourself into.

Not many people in my situation were so lucky, many of us don't get to live on, many of us hold on to life knowing that it is going to be taken away from a brain tumor. Many people in my situation are disabled, many lost sight in an eye, many became manic-depressive people and so many more became epileptics. Somehow, I escaped those things. I made it! I can think, reason, don't get irrational or do all of the things that could have happened. My feet work, my hands work, my mind works and I can see out of both eyes. Isn't that marvelous? I will never look at another person with scrutiny, but I will examine why they are and why they behave like they do. I won't judge you, I will wonder and ask questions because I want to understand.

If I had to do this alone, I would not have tried. I wanted to live for my husband and children. I wanted to know what being a senior citizen is like, I want to know what a long time marriage would be, I want to look at my husband, both of us old and frail with caring and loving eyes. A bit of a romantic in my soul, definitely. Obstacles that stand in my way are a challenge and tackling them is normally fun for me, this was one that wasn't. Remembering that intense fear of thinking I could die or be disabled was horrifying. Shaking with nerves was something that had to be put to bed. This book has done that.

Life is now a thing I grasp on to. Hold on to it tightly, enjoy life, look at it, and examine where you are going and where you want to be. Think about it, don't leap after risks, and always remember it could be the last time you get to hold on to it. Life, it's not something to abuse, we all need to use it.

I listen to people around me, I listen to the news and I listen to what you have to say when you talk to me. It's educational in some way and it's all something we have to share. If for one minute you listen to someone talking to you they have something you could use, make your own decision about and carry on from there.

There has been pain in so many things that happened along the road of "Hindrances" that I shared with you, a tiny part of my life that belongs to all of us. Survival, suffering and joy are a vital part of living that we don't even put it to that context when we live our daily lives until something threatens it.

From here on in, I am going to live my life. With my husband and children, and pets. They are important, just I am to myself. If anything you have read in this book, I will ask that you do one thing, enjoy your life. Smile, it hurts less when you do, be kind to yourself and the people you love. It does come back to you.

Printed in the United States
58432LVS00004B/280

9 781424 123124